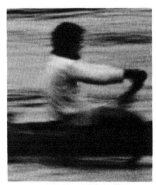

Row For Your Life

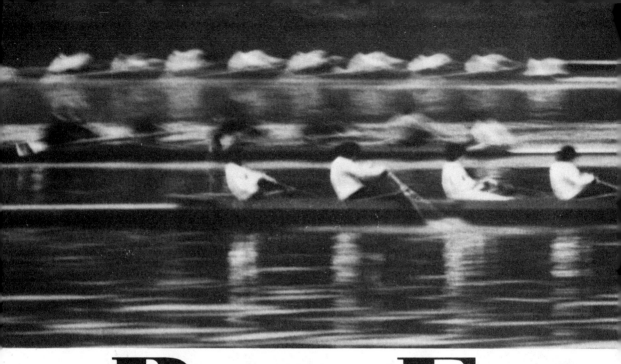

Row For

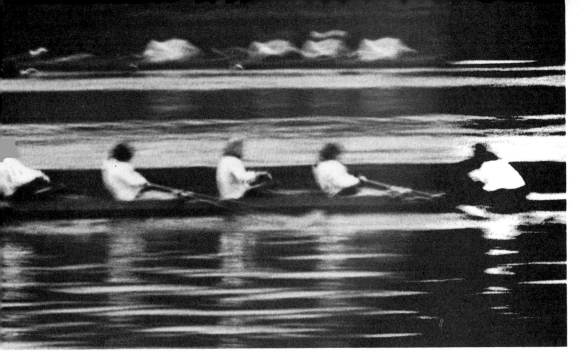

Your Life

*A Complete Program
of Aerobic Endurance Training*

by Barbara Kirch,
Dr. Reed W. Hoyt,
and Janet Fithian

Photographs by John Costello,
Eric Mitchell, and Susan Daboll
Produced by The QWERTY Group, Inc.

A Fireside Book
Published by Simon & Schuster, Inc.
New York

The Avita 950 Rowing Machine, used in some of the photographs, was supplied courtesy of

**The Fitness Depot
676 Broadway
New York, N.Y.,**

and we are thankful to Mr. Thomas Schneider and Mr. Thomas O'Brien for their cooperation and assistance.

Copyright © 1985 by The Qwerty Group, Inc.
All rights reserved
including the right of reproduction
in whole or in part in any form
A Fireside Book
Published by Simon & Schuster, Inc.
Simon & Schuster Building
Rockefeller Center
1230 Avenue of the Americas
New York, New York 10020
FIRESIDE and colophon are registered trademarks of Simon & Schuster, Inc.

Designed by H. Roberts Design

Manufactured in the United States of America
10 9 8 7 6 5 4 3 2 1

Library of Congress Cataloging in Publication Data
Kirch, Barbara.
   Row for your life.

   "A Fireside book."
   Bibliography: p.
   1. Rowing.   2. Physical fitness.   3. Aerobic exercises.
4. Exercise—Equipment and supplies.   I. Hoyt, Reed W.
II. Fithian, Janet.   III. Title.
GV791.K57   1985   613.7'1   85-15917
ISBN: 0-671-55447-6

Acknowledgments

The authors are indebted to many professionals in athletics, medicine, and fitness for sharing their knowledge, opinions, and experience.

We would like to thank Bruce Konopka, Head Coach, Women's Crew, University of Pennsylvania, for helping to initiate this project; oarsman David Krmpotich for insights into the sport of rowing; and oarsman William Donoho for research into available equipment.

Nurses, exercise physiologists, and physical therapists in fitness and rehabilitation facilities were especially helpful in providing insights about the use of rowers as a means to fitness and about equipment. Among these, personnel from the cardiac rehabilitation facilities at Crozier Chester Medical Center, Chester, Pa., and Bridgeton Community Hospital, Bridgeton, N.J.; Ed Miersch, M.A., A.T.C., Director of the Sports Medicine Clinic at Haverford Community Hospital, Havertown, Pa.; Jeanie Compesi, M.S., an exercise physiologist at Abington Memorial Health Services, Willow Grove, Pa.; and Thomas J. Suspenski, L.P.T./A.T.C., Program Director of the Sports Medicine Institute of Delaware County Memorial Hospital, Drexel Hill, Pa., were especially helpful and showed enthusiasm and dedication to their work. Joseph Vegso, M.S., A.T.C., Head Athletic Trainer, Sports Medicine Center, University of Pennsylvania, also provided much helpful information. Lipid researcher Dr. Paul Coates, Associate Professor of Pediatrics at the University of Pennsylvania, most generously reviewed the chapter on the effects of exercise on lipids.

We are especially grateful for the interest in the project by the United States Rowing Association. Christopher Blackwell and Kathryn Reith were generous in allowing the use of USRA files and in providing an awareness of the number and variety of people who make rowing a part of their daily lives. Dolly Driscoll's enthusiasm for and dedication to rowing was an inspiration and provided us with an appreciation of the value of rowing as a rehabilitative exercise medium.

Total Health Equipment of Pennsauken, N.J., provided us with equipment for trial and helpful comments on the advantages and disadvantages of various products. M. and R. Industries, Inc., and Concept II provided us with long-term use of equipment.

The authors also appreciate the assistance with the manuscript by Charles Griffin and Maria Hellman.

Finally, the authors would like to thank David Fay Smith and F. Joseph Spieler of the QWERTY Group for their assistance in developing the idea of this book.

To the memory of
John B. Kelly, Jr.,
a fine oarsman and a great
friend of amateur athletics

Contents

10 · ROW FOR YOUR LIFE

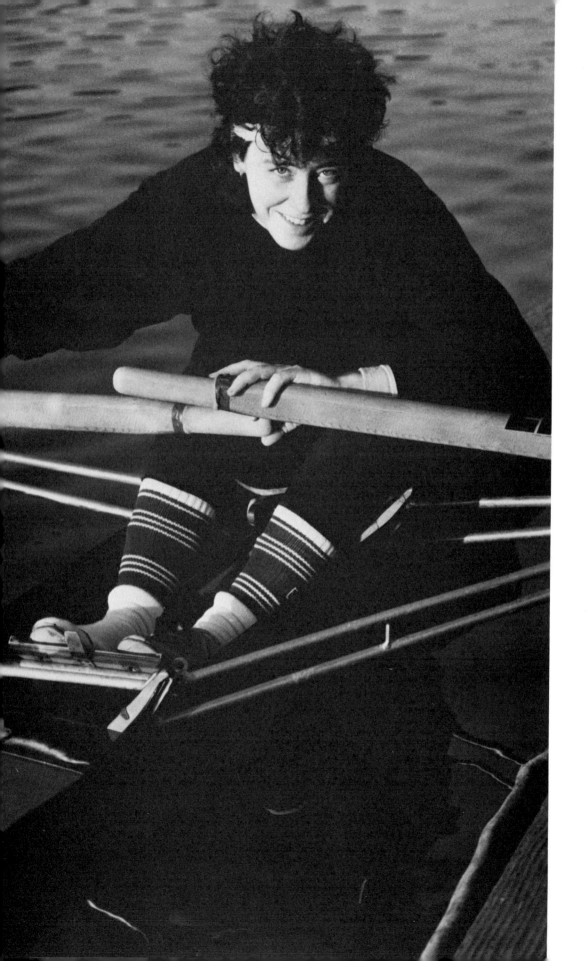

Preface

As an athlete, fitness is my first concern. I give many hours each day to it, for without strength and endurance I could not excel in rowing. But there are many reasons for staying fit.

Cardiovascular fitness is the most important reason and applies to everyone, young or old, whether or not you are or have ever been athletic. Fitness can be achieved without athletic skill. It merely takes a commitment to spend a few hours a week in a motion vigorous enough to bring the heart rate to a level where conditioning can occur. It is clear from medical research that fitness pays off in a healthier, more productive, and possibly even longer life. The training program we have devised is based on medically sound principles for cardiovascular conditioning and is appropriate, with modifications, for a variety of people.

Rowing is an excellent means to fitness. Whether on the water, in training facilities, or in people's homes, a variety of people are using rowing for conditioning and recreation. This is exciting. My own training includes work both on the water and off.

What fascinates me about rowing is that it requires a combination of strength, endurance, and skill. It was a breakthrough for me because I could distract myself from the pain and exhaustion of training for competition by concentrating on technique. Rowing is truly a full-body sport.

My most exciting moments in rowing come when I am so focused on making the boat glide forward that I don't even feel how hard I am pulling. I am being as powerful and explosive as I can, but I am also focusing on effectiveness, balancing on the fine edge between blind exertion and the right amount of concentration to keep my body under control. The boat feels like it is barely skimming the surface of the water. During moments like these, I want time to stand still.

I still don't like the pain that goes with my level of training, when my muscles scream for oxygen and switching from one breath per stroke to two doesn't satisy them. I dread the transition between aerobic and anaerobic metabolism that goes with finding this "second wind," but my body seems to perform almost automatically.

I have learned what many people have told me is true of all achievement. If you want something to happen, you must make it happen yourself. Dreams are nice, but someone has to make them a reality. And that someone is you, or me, with simple hard work. Fortunately, most people do not have to train the way I do to achieve better health and a stronger heart. You can do it with a few good workouts each week, and some careful measurements to show you the effects of your training. Here's how. . . .

Barbara Kirch

1

The Exercise Initiative

Physical Activity Is a Biological Need

Your body is not in simple equilibrium with your environment but is a dynamic, ever-changing system. A constant stream of energy passes through it to sustain a harmonious relationship between you and your surroundings. Exercise increases this flow of energy and can help bring your body and mind to a higher state of organization.

The human body is evolutionarily designed for strength and endurance. Although human intelligence is usually credited with man's success in adapting to changing and sometimes hostile environments, this success has only been possible because the human body was capable of carrying out ideas emanating from the mind. But within the last century, strength and endurance have become secondary attributes for survival. Most of us can now earn a living and take care of personal needs without the kind of effort that produces sweat, builds muscles, and makes the heart race. Yet we still have the physiology for exertion—the physiology that was so important for man's survival.

Living in a society that has become out of sync with our physiology has many expressions. There are feelings of malaise, stress, or free-floating aggression. There is dissatisfaction with the way the body responds when called upon for activity. Even those who are successful in their careers and personal relationships experience a sense of stagnation, of not physically achieving their potential.

The urge to exercise is probably primordial. Dance and sport have provided the natural highs for many cultures from early times. Gradually, spectator sports have become a popular means to satisfy this urge, but in recent years more and more people have found such secondhand experience unsatisfactory. Doing, not watching, is the thing. Statistics indicate that by the late 1970s, nearly half of all Americans were participating in some sort of physical exercise daily, double the number of that in the early 1960s. A fitness—or exercise—industry has sprung up in response. Gyms are as numerous as grocery stores. The exercise industry has its stars, literature, equipment, and entrepreneurs who are responding to a widespread feeling of unease and a determination to do something about it.

If you share these feelings and want to banish them, you must first overcome the negativity that accompanies inactivity. You may question whether exercise offers you benefits that are worth the trouble and can be achieved within your limited time budget. The evidence is convincing. You will look better, feel better, accomplish more, and get more out of life if you exercise. Further, these benefits can be yours for about an hour and a half a week—practically throwaway time.

An understanding of the numerous benefits of exercise that can be yours, no matter what your age or current state of conditioning, will help you overcome your negativity and push you toward increased activity. Energy will then begin to flow, and you will feel more creative and positive about many aspects of your life, including the decision to make endurance exercise an intrinsic part of your life.

Cardiovascular Fitness—
The Effects of Conditioning

Cardiovascular disease is the major cause of death in the United States. However, between 1968 and 1978 deaths from coronary heart disease (CHD) dropped 26.5 percent and from cerebro-vascular diseases, 37.7 percent. Major reasons for this decline have been a decrease in smoking, dietary changes, greater awareness of the importance of treating hypertension, and an increase in physical activity. Numerous scientific studies document the positive effects of aerobic exercise on the cardiovascular system and provide statistical evidence for a link between physical fitness and cardiovascular health.

The Effects of Conditioning on the Cardiovascular System—Here are some concepts that will help you understand the beneficial changes in the cardiovascular system that can be induced by endurance training, that is, by regular aerobic activity. In describing the benefits of exercise and designing an aerobic exercise program, it is necessary to consider:

- stroke volume
- heart rate
- cardiac output
- maximal oxygen consumption (VO_2 max).

Stroke volume refers to the amount of blood that the heart ejects with each contraction. When stroke volume increases, with each beat the heart puts out more blood to supply the body's needs.

Heart rate is the number of times that the heart contracts per minute. Heart rate and stroke volume are closely related. When stroke volume is increased, the heart does not have to contract as often to provide the body's tissues with sufficient blood. The heart rate both at rest and against a given work load lowers as stroke volume increases.

Cardiac output is the total amount of blood pumped per minute by the heart. This is determined by multiplying the heart rate by the stroke volume. Cardiac output is one indicator of the heart's capacity to put out enough blood to meet the various demands of life.

Maximal oxygen consumption (VO_2 max) is a measure of a person's maximal ability to generate energy with oxygen. It is also an excellent indicator of the individual's capacity for sustained heavy work. Maximal oxygen consumption depends on the rate of oxygen transport, which is in turn a function of cardiac output, the amount of oxygen carried by the blood, and the distribution of blood flow.

Maximal oxygen consumption decreases with age but this decline can be reduced through a lifetime of endurance conditioning. Some older athletes have a greater VO_2 max than much younger sedentary people. Just how high the VO_2 max can go depends on the training habits and the genetically determined characteristics of a person's cardiovascular, respiratory, and cellular metabolic systems. Increases in maximal oxygen consumption occur through increases in the rate of oxygen transport to the cells and increases in the tissues' ability to consume oxygen. The result is an increased ability to carry out heavy activity for long periods without exhaustion.

An endurance exercise program can increase stroke volume so that with each heart beat more blood is made available to the circulatory system. The increase can be very great. For example, the heart of a trained athlete at rest will pump out 40 percent more per contraction than that of a sedentary individual. Looking at it another way, a sedentary person's heart will have to beat 140 times to do what a trained athlete's heart will do in 100 beats. During exercise, the difference between the heart rates is as great or greater. In endurance trained individuals, stroke volume increases with the transition from rest to exercise. In untrained individuals, the stroke volume increases only slightly, requiring a very rapid heart rate to meet the body's increased metabolic demand for oxygenated blood.

A lower heart rate at any level of activity—indicative of increased stroke volume and improvements in the circulatory system—can be achieved with exercise in as short a time as three weeks. Sedentary people will see

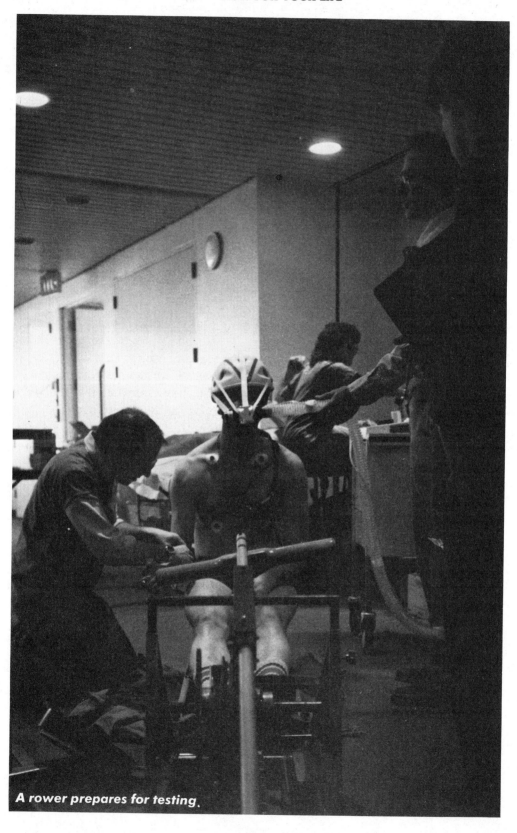

A rower prepares for testing.

improvement even more quickly than those who are already fit and are looking for signs of further cardiovascular improvement.

Not only does training enable the heart to put out more blood with fewer, more powerful contractions, it increases the amount of oxygen that can be extracted from hemoglobin and used by the tissues. As you know, hemoglobin is the oxygen-carrying pigment in the red blood cell. Training also increases tissue oxygenation by increasing capillary density in the working muscles. Increases in capillary density of 15 to 20 percent have been found to correspond to the increase of maximal oxygen consumption and blood flow to the legs after two to three months conditioning. In other words, people in training actually grow more capillaries, those tiny blood vessels where the transfer of oxygen to the tissues actually takes place. Conditioning over several years has resulted in capillary densities 60 percent greater than those in sedentary individuals. These changes add to the beneficial effects of training, allowing for an all-around more efficient system of providing the tissues with oxygen.

If you have been leading a sedentary life and begin exercising an hour or two a week at a sufficient intensity, you can realize benefits to your cardiovascular system within three weeks. To achieve the cardiovascular benefits of exercise generally requires three sessions per week at a heart rate of 130 to 150 for about twenty to thirty minutes, although lower intensity and duration may benefit older or very sedentary people. Some studies have shown two such training sessions to be sufficient. Detectable effects have even been found in response to vigorous exercise once a week or even running in place only twelve minutes daily. Positive effects disappear quickly, however. If exercise is stopped, your cardiovascular condition will regress to its former state within about three weeks.

That moderate amounts of exercise can remodel the cardiovascular system for greater efficiency is strongly supported by scientific evidence. But does this actually translate into good health and a longer life? There is very convincing statistical evidence that it does.

The Statistical Link Between Activity and Health

There have been numerous long term studies of the effect of an active lifestyle on the incidence of coronary heart disease (CHD). Since CHD is the main killer in our society, it makes sense to pay attention to the findings. The studies have covered periods of more than twenty years and have included groups as diverse as San Francisco longshoremen, London bus drivers, and Harvard alumni.

The overwhelming statistical evidence is that regardless of your age, weight, smoking habits, blood pressure, family history, lipid profile, or even prior heart problems, you are significantly better off with a program of regular exercise than without it.

The good news is that you can do something to improve your chances for a longer, healthier life, instead of simply taking what nature and habit seem to have selected. The even better news is that you don't have to do very much.

One of the largest studies is Dr. Ralph S. Paffenbarger's study of nearly 17,000 men who entered Harvard College between 1916 and 1950. These men are now in their fifties—and up into their eighties. The methodology of this study involved cataloging weekly activity patterns and measuring the caloric expenditures associated with such common activities as walking and stair climbing as well as various sports. Walking one city block per day, for example, uses 56 Kcal (calories) per week, while running spends 10 Kcal per minute.

The astonishing finding was that as little as 2000 Kcal per week of activity can make a major difference. Men who had expended fewer than 2000 Kcal per week in exercise were 64 percent more likely to experience coronary heart disease than those who had expended more than that. Interestingly, former varsity athletes who quit sports after college were at higher risk than nonathletes who took up and kept up some vigorous sports activity after college. A similar British study matched exercisers and nonexercisers on factors such as build, smoking habits, and family history, and found that fatal first heart attacks occurred 50 percent more often in nonexercisers.

The effects on blood pressure and hypertension are equally compelling. Any activity is demonstrably better than none, and vigorous activity is best of all.

Most of the long term CHD studies have been done on men, largely because men have had a much higher risk of heart disease than women. However, the studies of conditioning that have included women strongly document the cardiovascular benefits. Because those effects are similar for women and men, the conclusions of the larger studies on CHD risk should theoretically apply to women as well.

Smoothing Out Metabolic Peaks and Valleys

Regular aerobic activity has a positive effect on one's ability to adapt to stress. Endurance conditioning can result in improvements in metabolism—those chemical processes of the body by which food is broken down to provide energy and to establish or repair tissues.

When someone who is not used to dynamic activity is challenged by unfamiliar physical or emotional demands, the body's chemical response can be exaggerated. But physical training has been shown to modify this response. What follows is one illustration of how physical activity can improve blood glucose regulation and contribute to a smoother running machine with fewer metabolic peaks and valleys.

Glucose is a form of sugar and is a primary source of energy, present directly in many of the foods that we eat, and also produced by our bodies' processing of carbohydrates. The amount of glucose circulating in the blood at any given time is normally precisely controlled by the hormone insulin. Any excess glucose is stored in the body in the form of glycogen. As glucose in the blood is used up by either normal activity or exercise, stored glycogen is converted back into glucose—to provide more fuel, in effect.

A key fact is that the amount of glycogen storage available to you is limited. Also, as the store fills up, the space remaining becomes less accessible, like the higher shelves in a well filled pantry. It then requires more insulin to clear a given amount of glucose from the blood.

In endurance trained people, less insulin is needed to remove excess glucose from the circulation. Training enhances glucose tolerance during exercise and at rest. Glucose tolerance refers to the ability of insulin to effectively clear glucose derived from food from the circulation and store it for future use. When insulin cannot efficiently clear this glucose from the blood, blood sugar levels become abnormally high. Fluctuation in glucose levels can lead to undesirable fluctuations in mood and mental functions.

Levels of both plasma glucose and insulin vary less throughout the day in fit persons than they do in the unfit. Also, the levels of plasma insulin and glucose are lower after meals in conditioned individuals. Glucose values can return to premeal levels within thirty to sixty minutes after eating in trained subjects, but remain elevated two and a half hours after meals in untrained subjects. This is because physical activity enhances glucose removal from plasma, perhaps because of a greater cellular responsiveness to insulin. Physical training has been shown to reduce the insulin required to store away a given amount of glucose by 40 percent. It only takes one to three weeks of heavy or moderately heavy exercise to achieve such a response.

The increase in glucose tolerance seen with conditioning is also related to the amount of space available to store glucose in its storage form, glycogen. Activity makes this space available by partially depleting the existing supply of stored glycogen. When glycogen stores are high and space is not readily available, it takes more insulin to clear glucose from the blood.

Glucose tolerance can fall quickly, within three days of stopping endurance exercise if a high caloric intake is maintained. When an athlete stops training but maintains a high calorie diet, the glycogen storage space will quickly fill. Reducing caloric intake when caloric expenditure is reduced can avoid this situation.

There are many other ways that regular endurance exercise can improve metabolism. Some are still not very well understood, but what is clear is that a smoothly running hormonal and metabolic system is critical in coping with physical and mental stress.

Exercise Is a Means to a Better Lipid Profile

The risk of developing atherosclerosis and coronary heart disease has been associated with the levels of total cholesterol and triglycerides in the blood. Cholesterol, triglycerides, and other lipids are transported in the blood in particles called lipoproteins. Although cholesterol has become a bad word in terms of heart disease, it is necessary for life and is essential to the structure of all cell membranes.

There is an array of lipoproteins with differing compositions and functions. They are classified according to their density. Generally speaking, cholesterol is carried in three classes of lipoproteins. In an individual with a "normal" cholesterol level of 180 mg per 100 ml of plasma, the cholesterol would be distributed about like this:

100–120 mg (56–67%)	Low-Density Lipoproteins	(LDL)
40–60 mg (22–33%)	High-Density Lipoproteins	(HDL)
10–20 mg (6–11%)	Very Low-Density Lipoproteins	(VLDL)

Heredity, sex, diet, drugs, and lifestyle, as well as other factors not yet understood, affect not only the amount of cholesterol in the blood, but, perhaps more importantly, the distribution of cholesterol among the lipoprotein fractions.

High levels of cholesterol carried in LDL are associated with a high risk of atherosclerosis. On the other hand, high levels of cholesterol in HDL may actually have a protective effect. One current theory is that a major function of HDL is to transport cholesterol from the peripheral tissues, including cells in the arterial wall, where it causes so much trouble, back to the liver where it is either stored, reused, or excreted in the bile. High levels of HDL, thus, could help keep the arteries open.

A physician, when assessing the risk of heart disease for an individual, should consider the level of cholesterol in each lipoprotein fraction rather than merely the total cholesterol concentration in the blood. Such an analysis is called a lipid profile, and provides a more accurate picture of a person's susceptibility to heart disease.

In 1975, evidence was first published suggesting that low levels of HDL cholesterol are associated with increased risk of coronary heart disease. Since that time research on the relationship between the apparently beneficial HDL and heart disease has been intense. Factors that influence the level of HDL have also been sought. Women generally have higher levels of HDL cholesterol than do men of similar ages. In women, there is a slow but steady rise in plasma HDL cholesterol between the ages of twenty and sixty-five. There appears to be no such rise for men. Diet seems to have no effect on the levels of HDL in normal people, while moderate amounts of alcohol can lead to higher HDL levels. Smokers have higher levels of HDL than do nonsmokers.

For more than twenty years, reports in the scientific literature have associated an active lifestyle with higher levels of HDL cholesterol than found in the general population. Studies of men and women, young and old, and those with normal and elevated total cholesterol levels, have shown this tendency.

One such study contrasting male and female runners, aged thirty-five to fifty-nine, with less active control subjects, showed striking differences in HDL cholesterol levels. The mean HDL cholesterol for female runners was 40 percent higher than that for female controls. Male runners had a 49 percent higher value than did their less active counterparts.

The question arose as to whether factors aside from activity patterns could be responsible for the lipid profiles in either group. A more certain relationship between activity and HDL levels could be established if increased exercise could be shown to actually change HDL levels in individuals. To ascertain this, thirty-nine men underwent an exercise program that was vigorous, but not overly demanding. They ran five miles a week at an average of 7.5 miles per hour. At the end of the ten-week period, the proportion of cholesterol in LDL and VLDL had decreased significantly, and the proportion of HDL had risen significantly. This was the first study to show that increased activity could be responsible for the redistribution of cholesterol in lipoprotein fractions in what is considered a desirable direction. Another study of thirteen medical students who chose to either jog, cycle, or do calisthenics four times weekly for thirty-minute periods for seven weeks, showed changes of similar proportion.

An active occupation also seems to result in high levels of HDL cholesterol. For example, Finnish lumberjacks have significantly higher HDL cholesterol levels than do electricians in that country.

Elevated serum triglyceride levels are also associated with coronary heart disease. These are, however, reduced in active individuals. In the study contrasting the runners and the randomly selected controls, both male and female runners had triglyceride levels *half* those of the male and female controls. Previously sedentary individuals will also experience a beneficial lowering of triglycerides.

Even those considered to have normal triglyceride levels can experience a further beneficial lowering. Just as an active occupation can raise the HDL cholesterol levels, such an occupation can reduce triglyceride levels. This was seen with the Finnish lumberjacks and electricians.

Activity has also been shown to modify the difference in triglyceride levels between the sexes. Males in the general population have higher levels of triglycerides than do females, but male runners have shown higher levels of the protective HDL and lower levels of plasma triglycerides than sedentary women of the same age. Also, the considerable increase in triglycerides with age in the general population was not seen in male and female runners.

When total cholesterol is considered, not all studies show a meaningful reduction related to activity. But one study of 133 men who participated in a ten-week program of various activities did experience a fall in total cholesterol. The dynamic activities such as running and cycling produced this change, but static activity such as weightlifting did not. Because rowing is a dynamic activity, you should, with your rowing program, expect to see similar results.

How much exercise does it take to produce these beneficial effects? In a study of running in middle-aged men, beneficial lipoprotein changes were seen only in those who ran eight or more miles a week. Another, larger study divided into two groups 100 middle-aged men who were matched for body weight, VO_2 max, lipid levels, and habits relating to smoking and alcohol. One group was asked to remain sedentary. Those in the second group were allowed to choose a mode of exercise that pleased them. The activities chosen included walking, jogging, swimming, skiing, and cycling. For the first eight weeks they got used to the exercise program, which included a fifteen-minute warm-up, thirty-minute period of vigorous exercise, and ten-minute cooldown. Then they were to exercise at a specific heart rate. During this period of training, there was a progressive decrease in serum triglycerides and increase in HDL cholesterol. These changes were seen in all but three of the forty-four who completed the program and were not related to decreases in body weight. It is not unreasonable to suppose that greater positive changes would be achieved with a higher degree of training.

This research, and other work not cited, provide convincing evidence that mild to moderate physical activity lowers triglycerides and raises HDL cholesterol levels. In many cases, the level of exercise needed to produce these changes was similar to that which you can do on your rower. Your rowing program, the more active lifestyle that increased fitness will foster, and dietary discretion should result in a lipid profile that is favorable to cardiovascular health.

Weight Management

Exercise is definitely not an expressway to weight loss. This may make you want to put this book away and pack up your rower, but before you do, consider these points.

• Regular endurance exercise combined with calorie counting can be an effective way to gradually reduce your weight.
• Any individual, whether overweight or not, can derive important benefits from regular exercise, including an improved capacity for the heart to pump blood, a lower blood pressure, and a more efficient flow of nutrients. It is important to separate being overweight from being out of shape. The two do not necessarily go hand-in-hand.

If you are overweight, you know the frustration of trying to lose weight or the despair of having lost weight only to regain it. And you know the negative effect these failures have on your self-image. Why not try another tactic and focus away from food—either the food you do eat or do not eat—and toward activity?

Formulate goals aside from weight loss. One can be improved cardiac function and respiratory function. The improved level of function brought about by consistent endurance exercise will help you deal with life's day-to-day demands and enable you to participate in a variety of activities. In a short time, stairs will no longer be an obstacle. You won't want to wait for an elevator to go up two flights. You will walk instead of ride because you will no longer be as short of breath. This increase in activity will enhance your self-esteem, raise your spirits, and diminish your dependence on eating for recreation or out of frustration. The exercise program outlined in this book will not slim you down for the class reunion next month but it will improve your cardiovascular function so you can dance all night.

Another goal can be an improved appearance unrelated to weight loss. You've probably noticed that some active heavyset people look very nice. Your exercise program can produce similar positive changes in your appearance. Your muscles will be more taut, your body less flabby. Pounds may not pour off, but inches will creep away. You will move more gracefully and quickly. Your body will be a more comfortable and useful companion to the inner you, and you will begin to feel more like your more slender counterparts.

The improved state of mind and higher level of energy that will come from exercising regularly will help you formulate and reach other new goals in many areas of your life. So take a break. Forget about being fat, but remember to exercise.

Exercise and the Overweight

Overweight persons enjoy the same physiologic benefits from exercise as those of more ideal weight. Significant cardiovascular and metabolic benefits have been reported in overweight men and women who exercise. Among these are improvement in the body's ability to consume oxygen, a lower heart rate, and increased capillary density.

The risk of developing hypertension and heart disease in overweights can be greatly reduced by vigorous activity. This is strongly supported by the Harvard study. There was an association between being overweight and becoming hypertensive in men who did not exercise vigorously. However, this association was not nearly as great for active overweight persons.

Nonparticipants in vigorous sports activity who were 20 percent overweight had a 50 percent greater incidence of hypertension than their counterparts who were of ideal weight. In those who were 25 percent overweight, the risk jumped to 65 percent. But exercising strenuously for two hours a week reduced this risk by 25 percent. Four hours reduced it by 50 percent! Active overweight people also had a lower risk of cardiac heart disease than those who maintained a normal weight but did not exercise.

The English study that compared the relationship of the incidence of coronary heart disease to exercise also addressed the issue of the protective effects of exercise on overweight individuals. The two groups studied were men ranging from slim to obese and those who did and who did not exercise. The study brought to light two very interesting facts. One, that a lower rate of coronary heart disease was related to a lower body mass index. The other, which should encourage overweight people to exercise, was that when men of similar weight were compared, the incidence of heart disease was very much lower in those who exercised than in those who did not. Actually, those who reported no vigorous exercise and were of ideal body weight had a higher incidence of CHD than did the active overweights.

There are metabolic advantages to endurance training in overweight people, even if they remain overweight. With obesity, insulin does not have the normal effect in promoting uptake of glucose, resulting in an elevated level of blood sugar. However, training can promote a more efficient utilization of glucose in obese individuals as well as in persons of normal weight.

Weight losses through exercise alone are small compared to those that the seriously overweight person aims for by dieting. For example, in a study of ninety-five overweight men and women who actively trained for seventeen months, the mean decrease in body weight was 10.6 pounds for the men and 7.3 pounds for the women. Weight loss was concentrated in the first two months of the aerobic exercise program. Similar weight losses and the propensity to lose weight early in the program have been reported in other studies. Sometimes, though, no weight loss at all occurs.

A more successful tactic is combining diet and exercise by decreasing caloric intake and increasing caloric expenditure (exercise). How quickly and how much you lose will depend on what energy equation you set for yourself. Even small adjustments can be meaningful. For example, a reduction in daily food intake of 100 Kcal and an increase in daily energy output of 100 Kcal will result in the loss of twenty-one pounds of fat a year.

There are some other important advantages in combining diet and exercise for weight loss. Ideally, weight reduction should favor loss of fat over muscle mass. Unfortunately, weight loss by diet alone results in a significant loss of muscle mass. By combining diet with exercise, lean tissue is protected, with more of the weight lost being fat.

The nutrition section will teach you how to shift the energy-balance equation in your favor by making daily adjustments in food intake and energy expenditure. Weight reduction is a complex issue and many questions regarding obesity have not yet been answered. The incidence of failure to maintain weight lost through many dietary regimens is not encouraging and attests to the complexity of the obesity problem. It has even been suggested that periods of hardship throughout the history of humankind have encouraged the evolution of a metabolism that permitted fat to be stored against hard times. Today, in our society, the health hazards related to obesity outweigh the risk of starvation. Over the long term, a lifestyle that includes regular aerobic exercise and the reduction of about 1,000 calories from the diet each week may be the best solution to maintaining a healthy body weight.

Psychological Benefits of Exercise

The ancient Greeks—Hippocrates, Aristotle, and Plato—long ago declared that there was a close relationship between a physically fit body and a sound mind. Twentieth century science has confirmed that emotional reactions are closely linked to physiological reactions, although, amazingly, some scientists are still unconvinced of the psychological benefits of aerobic exercise. The difficulty in defining and measuring stress may explain why there is little hard scientific evidence that exercise relieves stress.

Does exercise enhance an individual's self-esteem and ability to get along with others? Scientific studies suggest that physical training often results in personal growth and success along with an improved self-perception.

A study of forty-five obese metropolitan policemen confirmed the correlation of an exercise-diet program with positive changes in self-concept. The subjects were divided into two groups. One received weekly educational sessions on nutrition and exercise. The other received the same instruction and participated in an aerobic conditioning program. Within eight weeks both groups showed improvement; however, those in the aerobic conditioning group showed two to three times more improvement in their self-satisfaction and personal view of their bodies.

Possible reasons for these positive personality changes include an increased state of physical fitness, an increase in the amount of energy for life, and a general feeling of well-being and competence. In addition they had the personal satisfaction of working with a group to achieve a fitness goal.

The psychological changes with endurance conditioning are paralleled by changes in the body's biochemistry. More oxygen is transported to the tissues, including the brain. Glucose and salt levels are better controlled, and changes take place in the levels of chemicals that control how nerve impulses are transmitted and received.

Flight or Fight and Anxiety—Anxiety and depression contribute to job absenteeism, suicide, heart attacks, alcoholism, and premature death. For example, 39 million Americans suffer enough anxiety and depression to alter their normal lifestyles. It is also estimated that anywhere from 30 to 70 percent of all patients seen by doctors are suffering from anxiety-related stress symptoms.

Anxiety, described as a feeling of apprehension, is often associated with an undesirable activation of the physiological fight or flight response. The fight or flight response is necessary in the presence of physical danger, when physical strength and agility are needed for self-defense or escape. Twentieth century citizens activate this response, not usually because of the need to escape some wild animal, but in response to the mental tension associated with modern living. The body, however, reacts to whatever is perceived, whether the threat is physical or mental:

- The muscles tense in anticipation of being used;
- A large quantity of adrenalin is pumped into the blood;
- Digestion ceases, as blood is shunted to the muscles and brain;
- The eyes dilate to allow more light to enter;
- Glucose levels in the blood rise to provide a source of quick energy;
- The heart rate rises to meet the increased metabolic demand for blood;
- Clotting mechanisms are activated to inhibit blood loss in the event of an injury.

This very sophisticated mechanism allows individuals to perform under extremely stressful situations, but the resulting state can be compared to that of an overpressurized steam boiler. If the pressure is not released, the boiler may develop stress cracks or blow up. Humans react in a similar way when the level of anxiety and tension exceed their capacity to cope. There is a feeling of being excessively charged up with all of the body's systems in a high state of readiness with no immediate form of release available. As a result, individuals can suffer from chronic disorders such as high blood pressure, and/or resort to excessive drinking, drug abuse, gambling, or even suicide.

Exertion is the natural final phase to the fight or flight response. Therefore exercise is a key means of relieving anxiety and tension associated with the fight or flight response. Numerous studies show that not only does vigorous exercise reduce anxiety, tension, and depression, it can be more effective than tranquilizers.

Exercise and Stress Tolerance—Endurance training can improve your ability to tolerate stress by profoundly affecting your metabolism. The very process by which chemicals are used to provide the energy and building blocks for life is altered. Biologically, the term "stress" refers to any physical, chemical or emotional factor that causes physical or mental tension.

Metabolically, your body responds to stress in a similar way, whether the stress is a result of heat, cold, high altitude, injury, surgery, or fear and anxiety.

The autonomic nervous system has a major role in regulating both the body's internal environment and its response to the external environment. The autonomic nervous system is divided into two distinct parts—one regulates the release of adrenalin and prepares the body for "flight or fight," and the other "digestive" part promotes the replenishing of energy stores and the repair of tissues. The autonomic nervous system is usually balanced—at certain times the adrenal side dominates, and at other times the digestive side dominates. Factors such as psychological stress, particularly in combination with a sedentary lifestyle, can upset this balance and lead to excess activity in the adrenal (flight or fight) side of the autonomic nervous system. These changes contribute to a reduced ability to tolerate stress, and an increased susceptibility to disease.

How much exercise is necessary to achieve an enhanced feeling of self and a reduction in your present level of stress? There is no definite answer. But programs such as those suggested in this book have been proven to decrease stress and contribute to a feeling of psychological, as well as physical, well-being.

Most important in deriving psychological benefits from a fitness program is to relax, approach the activity with enthusiasm, and let the good feelings come.

2

Why Row?

The human body, designed for activity, should be kept active. Exercise throughout life is beneficial to almost all bodily functions and structures. It is never too late to work toward a more active life. Now is the time to get down to work and achieve the personal fitness that can be yours.

The benefits of exercise can be achieved through exercise, work, or sports that involve steady, rhythmic activity employing large muscle groups and increasing the heart rate on a sustained basis. Such work can be done on a rower.

Your interest in the rowing machine as a vehicle for physical fitness indicates some awareness of the advantages of rowing as exercise. Perhaps there are other advantages that you had not considered.

Total Body Exercise—Conditioning Many Muscle Groups

Rowing provides more total body exercise than most other forms of exercise, except swimming and cross-country skiing. Done properly on a well-functioning machine, the rowing stroke uses major muscle groups in the arms, shoulders, back, stomach, and legs. Walking briskly, running, and cycling are all excellent means to build endurance, but they fail to utilize the muscle groups in the upper body. Upper body conditioning is beginning to be recognized as important. This is the impetus for the popularity of light weights used during walking, running, and dancing. An untrained upper body may not be able to respond when called upon to work, with resultant stress to the cardiovascular system. For example, a person conditioned through running or cycling may find his heart stressed when shoveling snow.

Although the primary goal of aerobic exercise—which is what you will be doing—is to build endurance, rowing also increases strength. The resistance presented by the pull is sufficient, with a high degree of repetition, to strengthen and tone muscles. On some rowers, the resistance is adjustable for strength conditioning. Both male and female rowers have beautiful legs and upper bodies as a result.

Because rowing uses both the upper and lower body, it is less boring and more challenging than exercise with other forms of equipment.

Rowing Meets a Variety of Special Exercise Needs

Most rehabilitation centers in hospitals include rowing machines in their array of equipment. In an informal survey of several of these centers, the physical therapists and rehabilitation nurses were enthusiastic about rowing as a means of conditioning their patients, themselves, and their families. Many had even purchased rowers for home use. As a group, they felt the machines were excellent for bringing the heart rate up quickly, were orthopedically safe, and were effective in exercising many muscle groups. Rowing has proven to be excellent therapy for cardiac bypass and post—heart-attack patients and even people with severe rheumatoid arthritis. Of course, programs for these patients are designed individually and are carried out under medical supervision. Persons with arthritis, heart disease, hypertension, or orthopedic problems should definitely consult with their physicians before they vary the type, duration, and intensity of their activity.

Some Cardiac rehabilitation and employee fitness centers don't recommend the use of rowers by those having a history of back problems. The staff of these centers feel that back injuries can be avoided by keeping the spine straight (the correct rowing motion on any type machine never requires that the lower back be bent). Susceptible individuals must exercise extreme caution when using rowers.

Rowing is a *non-weight bearing* type of exercise. This makes it particularly suitable for those with certain orthopedic or neuromuscular problems. For example, with arthritis, the muscles around the joints should be kept as strong as possible and range of motion should be preserved. Weight-bearing activities, however, stress the joints and can increase discomfort and damage. Because rowing is done sitting down, joints are spared stress. The injuries to the hips, feet, and knees that go with sustained weight-bearing activity such as running are not seen in those who row.

A Convenient Means to Fitness You Can Stay With

Any exercise program, to be successful, must be maintained. Conditioning is based on regular aerobic activity, done week after week, throughout the year. You may be physically tuned up in September, but by January the improvements in cardiovascular function will have disappeared if your schedule of activity is not maintained. Some researchers have reported detraining effects—that is, loss of the physiological benefits of training—within three weeks!

So, to get fit and stay fit you must utilize an exercise program that is in keeping with your total lifestyle and can be carried out year around. How you do this will depend on personal preference, time available, weather, the exercise facilities available to you, and your physical attributes. What is important is that three or four times a week you do some form of activity that can bring your heart rate up to a conditioning level suitable for your age or physical condition for periods of a half hour or more. The Row for Your Life Program will show you how to determine your conditioning heart rate and design an overall program you can stay with.

The convenience and feeling of well-being that rowing offers make it a perfect means toward personal fitness. An effective workout program can take place right at home, with no travel time, no membership fees, and no special shoes or clothing required. Such convenience will help you establish the habit of a fitness program.

Your Rower—an Adjunct to Your Fitness Program

You may be already committed to exercise. Perhaps you run or swim. Or you enjoy aerobic dance classes. Those excellent aerobic exercises should be continued if you enjoy them. But there may be times when you cannot run or swim. With a rower you can then maintain your aerobic capacity. Another possibility is that your present activity might not provide you with enough aerobic activity. For example, a weekly aerobic dance class will definitely add to fitness, but once a week is not enough for meaningful physiologic benefits. Rowing can give you those necessary additional workouts.

Participants in sports such as tennis, softball, and golf (without a cart) are in better condition than are those who forego sports altogether. However, these are not aerobic activities. They do not provide a continuous, sustained increase in the heart rate sufficient to produce a training effect. An hour and a half a week on a rower can provide this training effect. It will also provide the endurance and strength that will increase your enjoyment and possibly your performance of your sport. Not being as susceptible to fatigue will enable you to concentrate on technique and achieve a greater proficiency in the sport. Translated, this means the games you love to play will be more fun.

In other words, rowing can meet a variety of fitness needs. A rower can be a useful tool for exercise in people who are already fit, who are striving for increased fitness, or who have special health problems for which exercise is advised. The training program in this book is based on your heart rate; it will be effective for you no matter what your present level of fitness. Also, there is a special section describing the modifications advised for older people.

3

A Primer in Human Exercise Physiology

The Oxygen Transport System

With few exceptions, your energy flow depends on a plentiful supply of oxygen. Oxygen is used to keep the metabolic fires burning, just as oxygen from the air is used by an open fire—in the final step, oxygen is used to form carbon dioxide (CO_2) and water (H_2O). In contrast to the typical fire, metabolic combustion releases energy from foodstuffs in a highly controlled, step-by-step process.

Very small organisms, composed of just a few cells, can simply absorb oxygen from their environment. But most animals, including humans, are much too large to obtain oxygen in this way. They must depend on a circulatory system to transport oxygen from the environment and deliver it to the cells where it is needed. The circulatory system also delivers nutrients to the cells and removes waste products.

Regular endurance exercise is an excellent way to keep your oxygen transport system in good working order. This will reduce the likelihood of heart and lung disease, and minimize the age-dependent reduction in the maximum capacity of the oxygen transport system.

The Pump and Plumbing

At the center of the circulatory system is an extraordinary pump—the heart. Based on a typical resting heart rate of seventy beats, or contractions, per minute, the heart beats at least 37 million times a year. This hollow muscle weighs about a pound and is divided into two pumping chambers. To visualize the arrangement of the pumps, make a fist with your left hand and wrap your right hand around it. Your fist represents the muscular, high-pressure left heart which receives oxygen-rich blood from the lungs and pumps it into the cells throughout the body. Your right hand wrapped around your fist represents the less muscular, low-pressure right heart which accepts oxygen-poor blood returning from the body and pumps it to the lungs where carbon dioxide is released and oxygen is taken up.

Although both sides of the heart pump equal amounts of blood, the high-pressure left heart must work against a higher resistance to deliver blood to the entire body. In contrast, the low-pressure right heart, which only has to pump blood through the lungs, works against a much lower resistance and is therefore less muscular.

Through rhythmic contractions, the left heart sends oxygen-rich blood to the body's tissues via a system of vessels. At the cellular level, oxygen and nutrients in the blood are exchanged for carbon dioxide and other metabolic waste products. Simultaneously, the right heart receives oxygen-poor blood from the body and pumps it through the lungs to pick up more oxygen. Like the plumbing in a garden fountain, the heart, lungs and blood vessels form a recirculating system which constantly receives and dispenses the same fluid, in this case blood. This very efficient circulatory system not only delivers the oxygen and nutrients to cells, but removes waste products for disposal.

The heart is amazingly responsive to the internal and external demands placed on your body. Exercise, emotion, heat stress, digestion, anemia, body position, and level of fitness all change heart rate. The extent of these changes varies with the individual depending on sex, age, health, and the individual reaction to a variety of stimuli. In the Exercise Program section you will learn how monitoring resting and exercise heart rates can be used to reach and maintain your individual fitness goal.

Endurance exercise conditioning results in a wide array of changes which extend far beyond the heart. During endurance exercise the working cells have a greater need for oxygen, nutrients, and waste removal. In response to the increased demand for energy production, skeletal muscle cells increase their biochemical capacity to generate power. They also increase the concentration of pigments which take up and transport oxygen within the muscles.

In addition to a heart to pump the blood, and arteries and veins to carry it to and from the tissues, an efficient oxygen delivery system requires a network of capillaries. These delicate capillary meshworks serve as the final transfer point where nutrients and oxygen are exchanged for cellular waste products and carbon dioxide. In response to the demands of sustained aerobic exercise, these capillary networks grow into ever more intimate association with the muscle cells. This reduces the distance between any cell and a capillary, and makes it easier to sustain a high energy output.

The flow of oxygen and nutrients to the cells also depends on the amount of blood pumped out by the heart and the resistance to blood flow through the body. Normally, these factors are matched such that blood pressure is in a healthy range. Sometimes, however, blood pressure can become chronically elevated and lead to severe health problems.

Blood Pressure

Blood pressure is something everyone talks about, but why be concerned? You know your doctor is because he or she takes it even when you only have a sore throat. Perhaps you have wondered what those numbers mean.

The numbers that make your blood pressure indicate the amount of pressure exerted against the walls of the arteries as your heart beats. These numbers, expressed in millimeters of mercury (mm Hg), are important indicators of how much high-pressure work your left heart is doing when it beats, and how much pressure it is exposed to when it is relaxing between beats. It is important for the health of your heart to keep both numbers within a normal range.

The higher or systolic number is the blood pressure generated by your left heart during the active or contraction part of your heart beat. The lower or diastolic number is the lowest arterial blood pressure during the relaxed period between beats when the heart is not contracting. Systolic blood pressure is related to the peak pressure the heart is generating when it contracts, and the diastolic blood pressure gives an indication of the ability of the body's vessels to accommodate the blood ejected by the heart. A typical blood pressure for a normal 20-year-old is 120 mm Hg for the systolic blood pressure and 70 mm Hg for the diastolic blood pressure.

As the heart ejects blood it is doing two kinds of work: volume work and pressure work. To maintain a healthy heart, it is far better to have your heart do volume work, such as that associated with endurance exercise, than it is to do the pressure work associated with purely strength exercises such as lifting heavy weights.

When one strains to lift a heavy object the skeletal muscles contract forcefully, collapsing capillaries and sharply reducing blood flow, but the heart keeps pumping blood. As the heart strains against a high resistance to blood flow, the type of work done by the heart shifts toward less volume work and more pressure work. The red face of the person lifting the heavy load attests to a high blood pressure. In response to this increase in pressure work, the heart muscle grows larger but the pumping ability doesn't increase. These changes do nothing to increase your capacity for endurance exercise and may be harmful to your long-term cardiovascular health.

When you have high blood pressure it is like lifting weights all day long, day in and day out. The heart responds to this pressure load with an increase in wall thickness. This is a dangerous and insidious trend because it becomes more and more difficult for oxygen to be delivered to all the cells that make up the enlarged heart muscle. As the cells within the heart muscle become starved for oxygen they can disrupt the normal rhythm of the heart. This is a key reason why people with chronic high blood pressure have a greater risk of having a heart attack.

Endurance exercise requires that the heart pump a large volume of blood to meet the increased demand for oxygen. In this case the heart works against a very low resistance to blood flow—volume work is high and the pressure work is low. Once again, the heart responds to the type of demand placed on it. In contrast to the pressure load generated by weight lifting, which causes the heart to develop thicker walls but does not change the stroke volume (the volume of blood ejected with each beat)—endurance work results in a much larger stroke volume and little thickening of the heart walls.

Your blood pressure depends on cardiac output (i.e., how much blood your heart is pumping) and what the resistance to blood flow is through the tissues. Both these factors are controlled by the autonomic nervous system—that part of the nervous system that supplies involuntary muscles, the heart muscle, and the glands, and is involved in the control of involuntary actions. Often, the source of high blood pressure is not known. A current theory is that the autonomic nervous system becomes imbalanced, leading to a high resistance to blood flow through the tissues. This in turn may lead to an increased cardiac output at rest, a high peripheral resistance to blood flow, and high blood pressure. Regular aerobic exercise is thought to reduce the resting activity of the sympathetic nervous system, and lead to a reduction in blood pressure.

As pointed out in the previous section, a number of studies have confirmed that exercise has a tremendous influence on whether or not an individual develops hypertension. The growing consensus is that it is important for everyone to exercise aerobically on a regular basis, monitor blood pressure, and limit intake of salt, caffeine, and alcohol.

Taking Your Own Blood Pressure

You can take your own blood pressure with some easily obtained and inexpensive equipment, a cuff and pressure gauge and a stethoscope. Also, there are a number of all-in-one blood pressure testing devices now on the market. Actually, the best way to keep track of your blood pressure is to do it at home for yourself. There are two problems with depending on blood pressure measurements taken during visits to the doctor. Blood pressure is often elevated due to the stress of visiting the doctor. Also, even if the measurement is accurate, it only represents a single moment in time. It is far better to regularly measure your own blood pressure in the relaxed environment of the home.

First of all, find a partner to practice with, preferably someone who knows how to take blood pressure. Have the person sit upright in a comfortable, relaxed position with his/her arms at the side. Wrap the blood pressure cuff snugly, but not too tightly, around the midportion of the upper arm. Gently place the bell of the stethoscope next to the artery in the crook of the arm, just below the cuff.

Quickly increase the cuff pressure until you are above the systolic pressure (about 160 mm Hg) and the artery collapses. No sound will be audible. Next, open the valve and gradually lower the pressure in the cuff. The first sound you hear as the pressure in the cuff decreases will be a hard thumping sound as blood first begins to squirt through the previously collapsed vessel. Look at the dial to read the systolic pressure. As you continue to lower the pressure in the cuff you will come to a point where the sound becomes muffled and quiet. Look at the dial again. This reading is termed the diastolic pressure. After completely releasing the pressure in the cuff, repeat the measurement again until you are confident of the results. Although 120 mm Hg systolic and 70 mm Hg diastolic, sometimes referred to as "120 over 70," is the ideal blood pressure for a young person, blood pressure increases with age, and at different rates for men and women, so check with your physician for an appropriate figure for you.

4

All About Rowing Machines— and the Right Way to Row

Rowing machines have undergone a dramatic transition from the costly and cumbersome ergometers found in boat house "dungeons" to more refined machines practical for home and institutional use. The use of rowers in homes, health clubs, and rehabilitation centers has grown explosively, and retailers report that rowing machines are their fastest selling fitness product. Manufacturers are continuing to refine current machines and develop new ones that will be more compact, reasonably priced, and that will more closely mimic the action of rowing a real boat.

There are two main groups of rowing machines or ergometers currently on the market. (1) Hydraulic cylinder type: the resistance comes from pulling against a hydraulic cylinder and (2) Straight-pull machine: a flywheel braked by a fan or a belt or an electrically braked motor provides the load. There are also less common and generally less expensive machines where the resistance is generated by friction. The hydraulic and straight-pull machines each have advantages and disadvantages, but both can be used for rhythmic, multiple-muscle, endurance exercise.

Currently, the most popular rower for the at-home exerciser uses hydraulic cylinders to create the load. This machine is commonly used in cardiac rehabilitation centers and is found in some health clubs. It is compact, easily stored, and quiet during operation. The simple design makes it less expensive than the straight-pull type described below. These machines, however, vary greatly in the sturdiness of construction and the action of the hydraulic cylinders.

There are a number of different rowers that use the hydraulic cylinder. Some have double-jointed pivots at the base of the oars which allow a wider range of motion and permit a variety of muscle groups in the upper back and arms to be worked. Others have inclined tracks that allow an easy recovery. In fact, rowing shells usually have seat tracks that are pitched to help on the recovery. It is important during an intense workout to relax on the recovery and allow blood flow to flush out the waste products and lactic acid. Most physical therapists who work with various machines feel that the hydraulic rower places more of a load on the back and arms than the flywheel machine does.

All hydraulic rowers use a similar system to generate the load. The amount of resistance depends on where the hydraulic cylinder is clamped onto the pivoting arm. If the cylinder is clamped near the base of the lever, the rower will have a large mechanical advantage and experience a light load. As the hydraulic cylinder is clamped progressively higher on the lever arm, the load will rise rapidly. The mechanical configuration makes it easy to set too high a load for low-load, high-repetition, endurance exercise.

A popular hydraulic model— the Avita 950 Professional Rower.

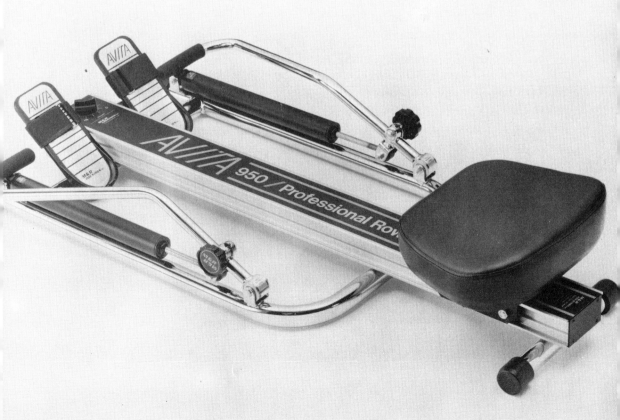

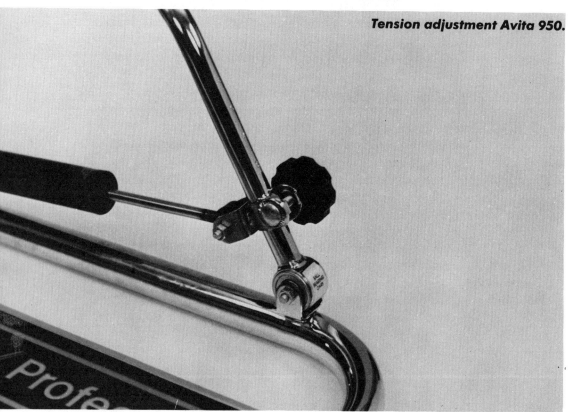

Tension adjustment Avita 950.

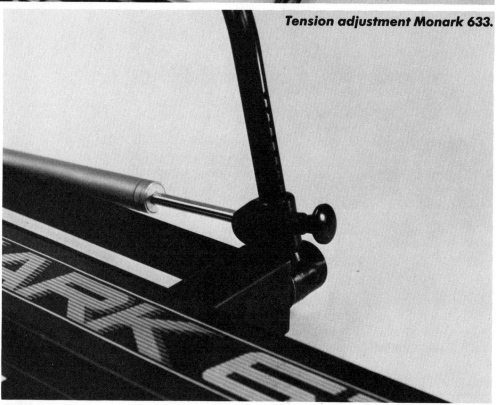

Tension adjustment Monark 633.

Some cylinders are, unfortunately, engineered so that at light resistance settings, there is no drag until well into the pull. This is a problem during the high-repetition, low-load situation of an endurance program. It is during the first portion of the pull that the legs should work to assist the arms in pulling back the oars. If there is no drag during this first phase in the stroke, then the leg muscles are not used. Most higher quality rowers have alleviated this problem by providing gas-assisted cylinders on their rowers.

In the straight-pull rowing machine, the load can be varied by changing the mechanical advantage relative to the flywheel or by varying the resistance presented by a band brake or an electrical braking system.

Straight-pull machines are more complex mechanically than the hydraulic types, and generally more expensive, but are highly popular with competitive oarsmen because they more accurately model the rowing of a shell. Most hydraulic machines require the hands to go through a single arcing motion, which does not affect the quality of the exercise; however, good technique in an actual rowing shell requires that the hands move in two horizontal planes: the drive plane, when the oarsman pulls against the oars buried in the water and the recovery plane, when the oarsman moves back to the initial compressed or "catch" position with the oars "feathered" out of the water.

AMF Benchmark 920.

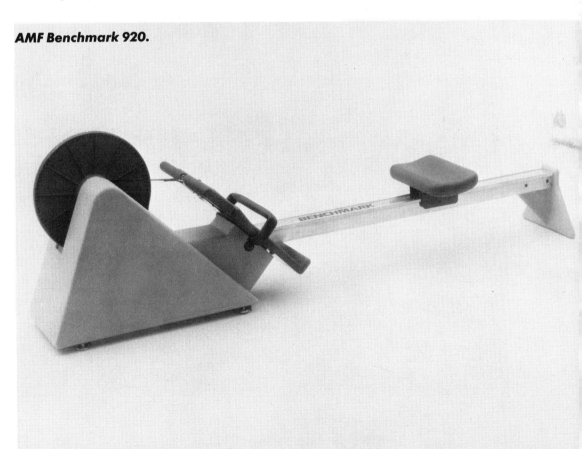

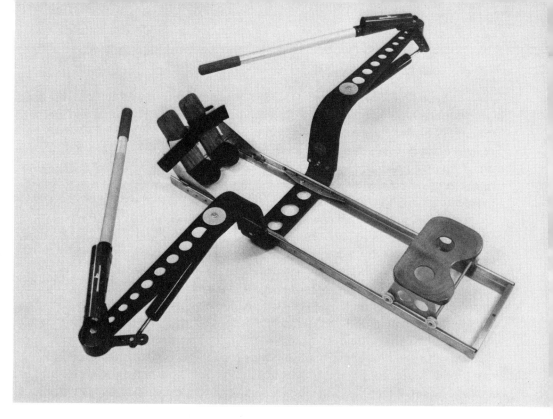

Martin Marine's "Oarcizer."

Martin Marine's "Oarmaster."

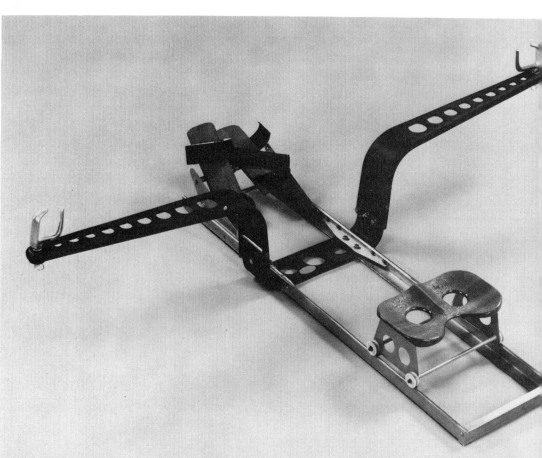

One hydraulic based machine that reproduces this action quite accurately is called the "Oarcizer®," made by Martin Marine. Actually, it is an accessory to this company's "Oarmaster®," a combination sliding seat and rigger/oarlock unit that fits into Martin Marine's Alden line of recreational shells and some other boats. The Oarcizer® attachments substitute for the oarlocks, and a pair of tubular aluminum handles for the oars. If you have an Alden for recreational rowing, the Oarcizer"® will enable you to use the Oarmaster® for exercise in the off season; but it is an expensive combination if you do not intend to row, too.

Competitive oarsmen also prefer the feel or "load" created by a fan-braked flywheel because it models the "run" (acceleration and deceleration) of a shell. In these machines, with the fan generating the drag, the rapid increase in resistance with fan speed is similar to the rapid increase in resistance experienced when trying to accelerate an actual shell. In contrast, a flywheel with a band brake, an electrically braked system, or a hydraulic system all have a more gradual increase in resistance.

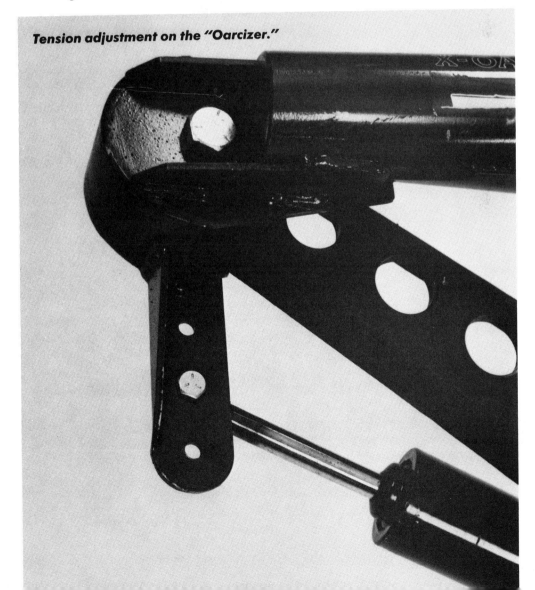

Tension adjustment on the "Oarcizer."

Exercisers as well as competitive oarsmen enjoy the sensation created by a flywheel machine. The fins on the moving flywheel create a refreshing breeze which adds a sense of action, even motion, to the workout. The rhythmic, swishing sound is also exhilarating, as is the smoothness of the rowing resistance and the pleasant recovery. The disadvantages of this machine to the average person are its size and cost. Some people might object to the noise. The unenclosed flywheel is dangerous for families with pets and small children. Nevertheless, the popularity of this type of machine, especially the Concept II (pictured), has risen to the point that there are ergometer races held in various cities throughout the winter.

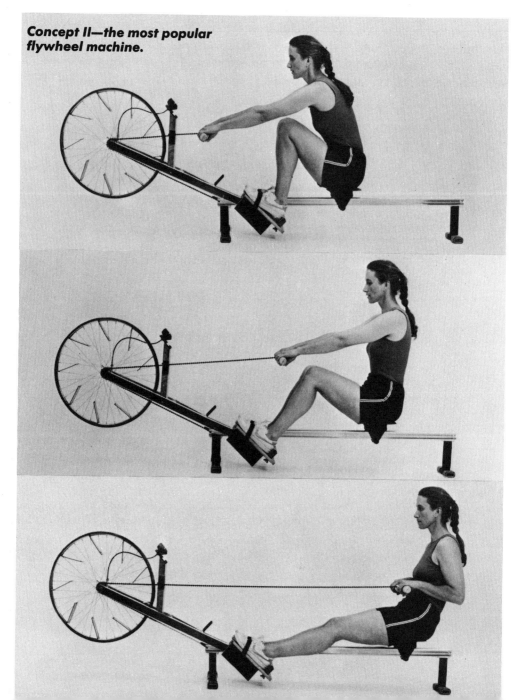

Concept II—the most popular flywheel machine.

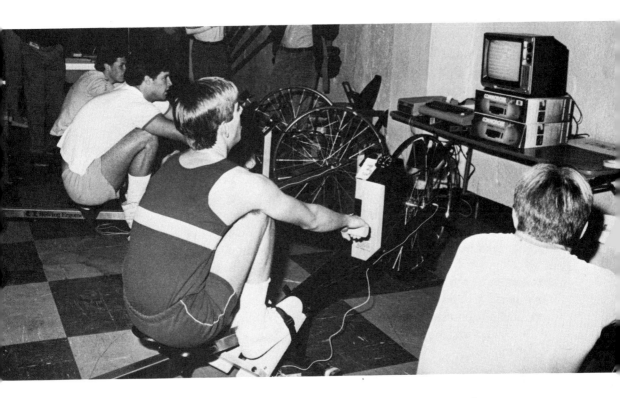

Concept II machines integrated with computer to simulate a real race.

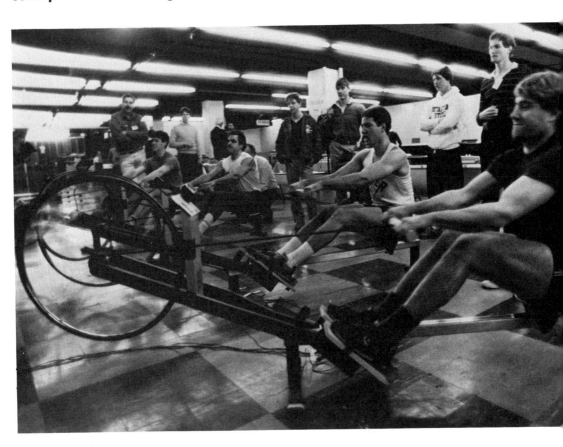

Choosing Your Machine

Rowing machines are available from a variety of firms, but the best place to try one out is an establishment that specializes in fitness equipment. Trained salespeople can point out the differences between the machines and help you decide which one fits your body and your needs. It is important to try a variety of machines because, unlike a bicycle, nothing except the load is adjustable. In your shopping, it may be difficult to find a straight-pull machine, but they are worth checking out.

When shopping, dress for exercise. Comfortable clothing and shoes will let you be at ease while giving the machine a good workout. Try the machine for several minutes. You should be prepared to raise your heart rate to 110 beats per minute or more and to work for at least ten minutes. Rowers will vary in noise level, so be sure to choose one you can live with. When you're finished, don't just ask yourself if you would want to continue on for another twenty, but whether the machine interests you as a daily companion in your long-term fitness program.

Orthopedic Considerations

From an orthopedic point of view, the ideal rowing motion is a horizontal "flat on your back" squat. Such a position would relieve the load on your back. The goal is to pull the weight of the oars as you would pick up a heavy load. When you pick up a heavy object you stand close to it, face it squarely, keep your lower back straight, and lift from a deep squat. The rowing machines in which the seat and foot rests are nearly at the same level begin to approach this configuration. In contrast, rowers that have a high seat position relative to the foot position will place a greater load on your lower back. Some, especially older people, prefer the higher seat model because they are easier to get on and off. There is obviously a tradeoff between features, but use extra care if you choose a higher seat model.

When considering a hydraulic rower, the fit between you and the machine is important. Try several on for size because you must be comfortable enough to work on the machine for periods of a half hour or more. You not only have to find a machine that works to your satisfaction, but one that fits your body. Is the machine long enough or short enough for you? Will the machine be big or small enough for all members of your family? Can you sit with your feet strapped in place and legs fully extended and not hit the end of the seat slide?

Do your feet fit in the foot plates? Are the foot plates arranged so that you can come forward on the slide until your shins are nearly vertical? In the hydraulic machines, the foot plates should have a cup for the heel, not just a bend in the metal. Foot straps should be easy to adjust, and if Velcro® is used

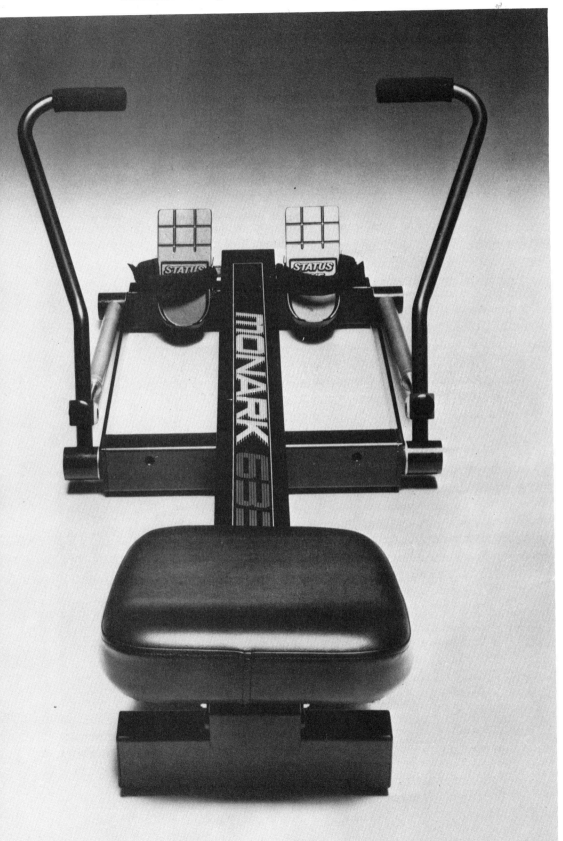

there should be enough to prevent slippage. Also, swiveling foot plates are superior to fixed foot plates. Try the straps. Is the arrangement convenient or would you find strapping in irritating every time you used the machine?

Does the machine operate smoothly, without squeaks and strains? Does the machine have ball bearings? Can the load be easily adjusted for comfort and challenge? Is the load constant at a given setting? There should be consistent resistance throughout the stroke at low, intermediate, and high settings. When you work at a high intensity, is the operation as smooth as it is at a lighter pace?

Do the oars extend far enough forward or backward to give you a full workout? Do they travel at a comfortable height and move smoothly or are there a lot of glitches?

Does the seat move freely, evenly, and quietly? Are you comfortable on the seat or do you slide around? A hard seat that provides proper support can be as comfortable as a soft one.

The machine should not be too heavy for you to handle easily if portability is a factor. A machine that can be easily lifted by a 6'2", 190-lb. man might not be so portable for a 5'2", 120-lb. woman.

Durability is another factor. A welded aluminum or welded chrome steel frame is preferable to the painted steel, bolted together frames on the cheaper models. A bar beneath the cylinder is advantageous because it prevents the frame from flexing or walking. The machine should not be susceptible to rust from sweat and dampness. Does the machine look sturdy? Does it flex and bend when you pick it up? To find out how a certain brand holds up, talk to friends

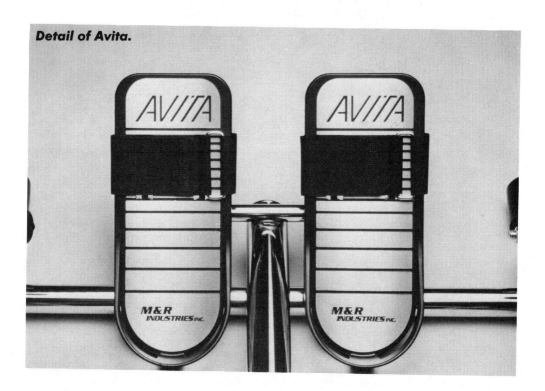

Detail of Avita.

and employees of fitness clubs and rehabilitation centers. Beware of low-quality imports or "knock offs," which may look legitimate, but don't have mechanical integrity. A five-minute phone call could save you hundreds of dollars and the chance for a really satisfying fitness program with a rower.

Remember, a rowing machine should be a rowing machine. Combination machines—that is, those that are also set up for bench presses, etc.,—are seldom bargains. In some cases, these peripheral devices compromise the function of the machine as a rower and they always add to the cost. Your money will be better spent, and you can develop a more satisfactory rowing program, if you choose a rower solely on the basis of the one primary function—rowing. However, there are non-rowing exercises that can be performed on a "pure" rowing machine. See pages 66–70.

Price cannot be ignored. You get what you pay for and cheap machines are a disaster! Consider several machines within a given price range. You can assume that two machines in the same price range will vary in a number of subtle and not-so-subtle ways. Single cylinder machines are generally not worth considering. Don't try to save $50 and buy a machine that you won't be happy with and therefore will not use. You are making an investment in yourself as well as in a piece of equipment.

You should enjoy using your fitness equipment. And it's a good bet that if it is not enjoyable to use, you will not use it. Perhaps you already have a fitness product or two stashed away in your basement ready for a yard sale. You certainly don't need another. There are enough machines on the market that you can probably find one that fits your needs and your pocketbook.

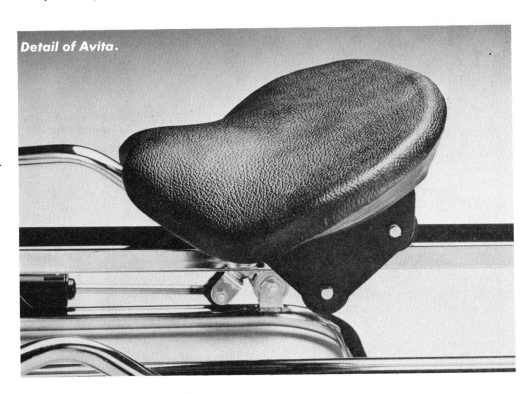

Detail of Avita.

The Avita 850—a model with a relatively high seat.

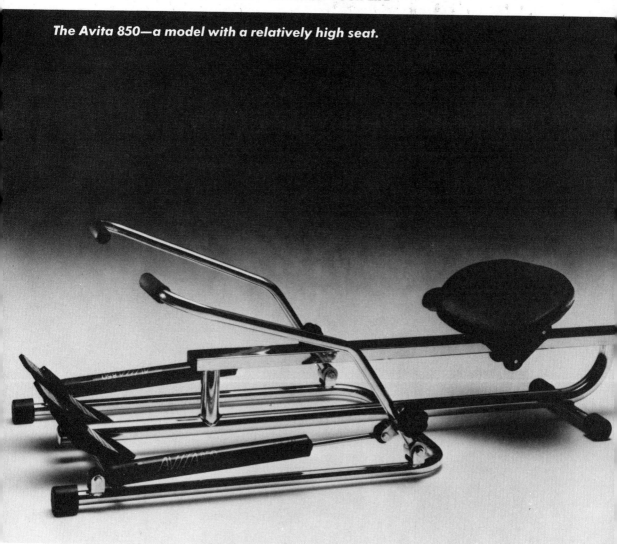

Accessories

Rowers also offer some high tech options, among them stroke meters and computers that give an estimate of work output. These options are costly and should not be the primary way that you monitor your performance. The important part of measuring any workout is heart rate and time. If you learn about your heart rate, meters won't be needed. If you do decide you want a computer or stroke meter for entertainment, make sure it is well sealed against your sweat and that it is of good enough quality to last for the machine's lifetime.

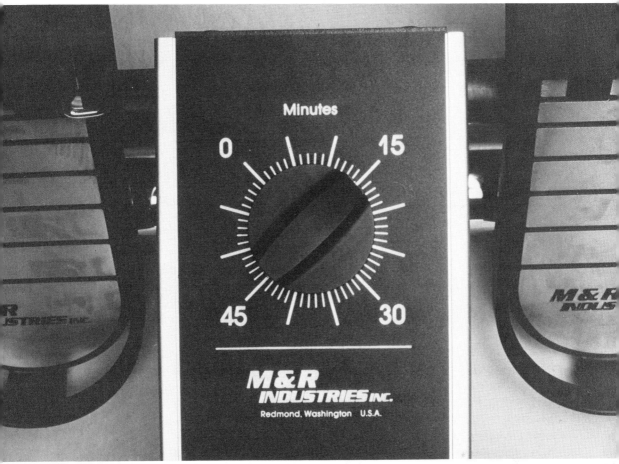

Detail of Avita.

Pulse monitors are a useful if somewhat expensive addition. There are a variety available. Not all work well during exercise. The most dependable type places the electrodes directly against the chest; the least dependable attaches a sensor to the end of the finger. Some monitors simply display the heart rate. More sophisticated ones may include a high and low heart-rate alarm, which acts as a reminder that you are either not working at a high enough intensity or are working too hard for your age or physical condition. Another useful feature is a clock which indicates the amount of time spent in the chosen heart rate range.

In a particularly dependable and convenient system made by AMF, the electrical signals from the heart are picked up by chest electrodes and sent by a miniature radio transmitter to a wrist watch monitor. The monitor then displays the heart rate and has a high and low alarm, as well as the capacity to record and play back the heart rate over the course of a workout. It even interfaces with a microcomputer.

Using the Machines

The top series shows Barbara Kirch on the Avita 950 hydraulic machine. The lower series shows Barbara on the Oarmaster® unit of an Alden

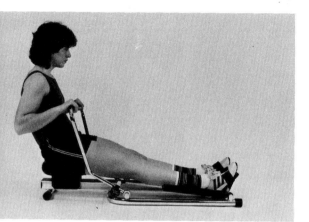

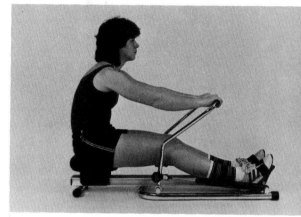

1. Many rowers start rowing from the Finish or runout position of a stroke. On the water, the blades would be flat to help stabilize the boat when it is not moving. We recommend that you begin your pattern the same way, on either kind of machine. Legs are all the way extended but knees are not locked. Hands are pulled close to the stomach but not touching it or not pulled past it to the sides if on a hydraulic rower. Locking knees at the end of a stroke can lead to knee injuries, and pulling the oars or handles past the plane of the stomach puts unnecessary strain on the lower back without adding much to the force of the stroke.

2. Begin your Recovery by curving your back slightly and extending your arms forward until your hands pass over your knees. Legs are still extended. On the Oarmaster® and in regular sculls, the convention is for the left hand and oar-handle to pass over the right. On hydraulic rowers, the hands stay parallel.

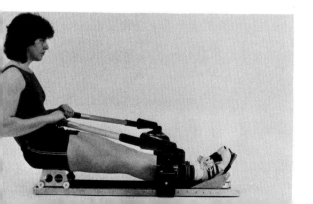

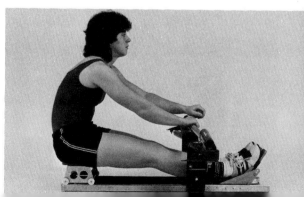

recreational shell equipped with the X-Oarcizer® attachments, demonstrating the correct form for rowing the machine or the actual shell.

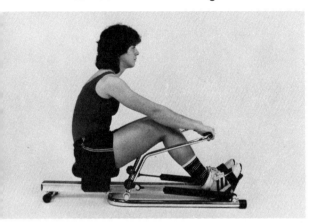

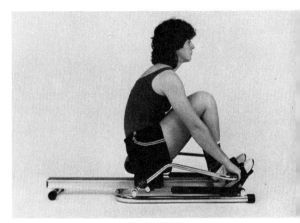

3. After your hands have cleared the tops of your knees, slide the seat smoothly forward so that your knees rise between your arms. Keep your head up and eyes forward. It is astonishing how quickly a tilt of the head can change the balance of a shell, and you may as well learn habits that will keep you upright when you go out on the water. In this phase of the stroke, form is nearly identical for both kinds of machine.

4. Stop the slide when your shins are nearly vertical and your knees are tucked against your chest and the insides of your arms. Keep your weight centered over the seat and don't let your bottom slide farther forward than your center line. Whether this particular error is even possible depends on the design of your machine and also of yourself. Avoid it because it puts extra strain on the lower back. Note that in a shell, the arms are extended and the hands are more or less over the toes, whereas on this hydraulic rower, they are down close to the ankles. Apart from the angle of the arms, the position of the body at the Catch is nearly identical on both rowers.

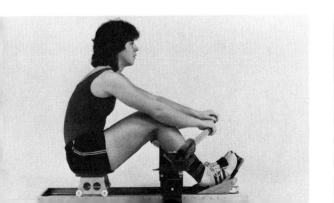

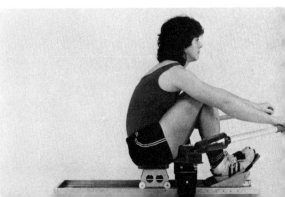

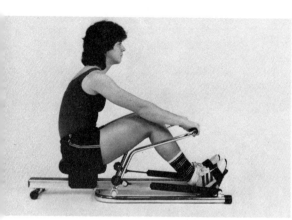

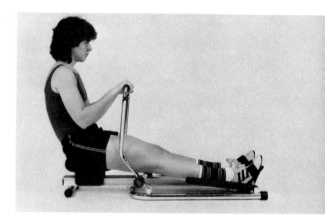

5. The Catch is when the oars dip into the water and the stroke begins. The power for the first part of the stroke comes from the legs. Keeping your arms straight, begin straightening your legs. Your back keeps its slightly curved posture and the seat slides back under your still-centered weight. Keep your head up and your eyes forward and level throughout the stroke.

6. When your hands are just about over your knees, start to open the angle between your back and legs by quickly swinging your shoulders back. Your arms are still straight, but the elbows should not be locked. Your arms pull in at the last minute, after your legs are fully extended (but not locked). Barbara is slightly more extended on the hydraulic machine in this phase because of the different geometry of the oars.

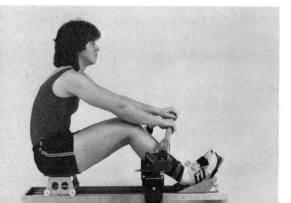

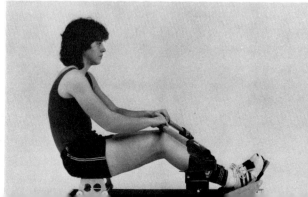

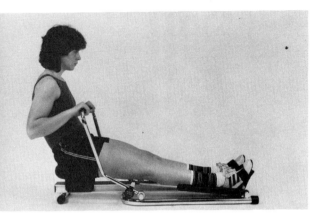

7. The arms and back provide most of the force for the Finish of the stroke, but the angle between legs and back should never open very wide. The force of the stroke comes from legs, shoulders and arms, in that order, while the back is curved but fairly rigid. The motion is similar to that of picking up a heavy object or doing deep knee bends, but in real rowing there is somewhat more curve in the back. If you feel any strain on your lower back, stick with the straighter profile. Pause very briefly at the finish, as if to let the boat run out, and then repeat the cycle, concentrating on smooth, fluid, consistent form rather than on sheer power.

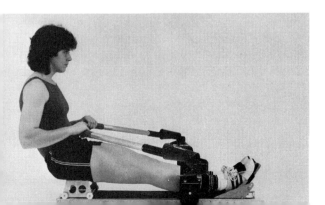

5

The "Row for Your Life" Program

Preprogram Check-up

Physical therapists and cardiac rehabilitation specialists are enthusiastic about rowing as a means of exercise for many of their patients. This attests to the safety and suitability of rowing for so many people. But it should be remembered that in rehabilitation centers, people with hypertension, heart disease, and other health problems carry out their rowing program under the supervision of trained health-care personnel. Such a safety net is not available to you, on your own, at home.

A sudden change in activity patterns, particularly those that stress the cardiovascular system and musculature in unfamiliar ways, can provoke some unwanted health problems. This is why a pre-exercise exam is recommended. A physician knowledgeable about and interested in exercise, or a sports physiologist, can guide you into a conditioning program suitable for your age and health and provide some supervision along the way. The combination of your desire for increased fitness, your physician's or health professional's interest in your health, and your exercise program may be just what is needed to spare you future cardiovascular problems.

Unfortunately, not all physicians are interested in exercise. Ask your physician if he or she is interested in doing an evaluation complete enough to give you the green light for some unfamiliar activity. Also, ask what the workup will include. If an exercise stress test isn't mentioned, the evaluation may not be worth your time or money.

An exercise stress test monitors your electrocardiogram and blood pressure during progressively more strenuous exercise, usually on a graded treadmill or a bicycle ergometer. This test tells how your heart reacts to strenuous activity and screens for heart disease too subtle to be detected by an ordinary resting electrocardiogram. It can also reveal the maximum exercise intensity (heart rate) to which you can subject yourself without danger.

Chances are, your heart will be capable of meeting the challenge of your fitness program. But if the stress test shows abnormalities, you should work with a cardiologist to define an exercise program suitable for you. It's also important to control your blood pressure, watch your diet, and break the smoking habit, if you have it.

Your musculoskeletal system should be evaluated. Don't fail to discuss with your doctor any back problems you have had. Generally, rowing is not indicated for people with a history of serious back problems.

If your physician seems uninterested in an assessment of your health as it relates to exercise, contact a sports medicine clinic. These can be found in most medical centers or in hospitals associated with medical schools. There, physicians will have the equipment, time, and interest in evaluating your health and the exercise program you are planning. Appendix B lists many sports medicine centers around the country.

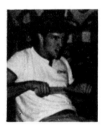

Four Fitness Elements

There are really only four elements in any cardiac fitness program. They are:

- Measurement—tracking your progress
- Intensity
- Duration
- Frequency

All the rest is pattern, embellishment, and variation. These are important, too, but the four main elements are critical. Of the four, the nonconditioning element, measurement, might just be the most important because it tells if the other three are doing the job of improving your fitness.

To work safely, effectively, and conveniently, a fitness program must be tailored to the individual. Decisions about how you train should reflect your age, present level of fitness, time constraints, and the type of exercise you choose to do. The best gauge of your condition is your own heart, and this program is based on that central idea. Your heart will tell you what kind of shape you are in now, and it will keep you informed about your progress.

As you now know, after a period of endurance training, the heart pumps out a larger volume of blood with each beat. This is referred to as an increase in stroke volume. Also, training changes the way your nervous system controls the blood supply to the skeletal muscles to permit more oxygen to be extracted from your blood. In other words, your heart and circulatory system become more efficient with exercise so that at rest or at any given load the heart has to beat fewer times per minute to supply your body's needs. By regularly measuring the changes in your heart rate at rest and at specific loads you can accurately follow the progress of your conditioning program and the performance of your oxygen delivery system.

The Reference Workout

Almost any regular exercise will give you a sense of well-being, but unless your oxygen delivery system becomes more efficient as measured by your reference workout, you are not getting the real benefits of working out. A reference workout simply measures your heart rate at three specific, reproducible workloads. By carefully controlling these factors and by doing your reference workouts at the same time of day, you can get a reliable indication of the effectiveness of your program.

A reference workout can be done with any form of exercise, such as bicycling, running, or rowing. But because you are attempting to gauge a rowing program under controlled conditions, use your rower. Here is a sample reference workout to use on your rower. Before you do one "for real," give this a try to see if it is difficult enough to challenge you (that is, to bring your heart rate up to training range) but not so difficult that you cannot finish the three phases without complete exhaustion. Because the program we are outlining is an aerobic one—that is, a high-repetition, low-load workout—the recommended load settings will range from low to medium. Higher settings will tend toward building strength, which is not the purpose of the program. If you want to make your reference workout more challenging than the one given here, increase the stroke rate rather than the load setting. Arrange your rower so that you can see a clock with a sweep second hand. Digitals are not as easy to read if you are already counting strokes.

Decide on three load settings on the rower and three corresponding stroke rates: that will result in heart rates between 60 and 85 percent of your maximum heart rate (220 − age). For example:

- 5 minutes at 30 strokes per minute on setting 1 or the lowest setting on your rower. (5 strokes/10 sec.)
- 3 minutes at 24 strokes per minute at setting 2. (4 strokes/10 sec.)
- 2 minutes at 18 strokes per minute at setting 3. (3 strokes/10 sec.)

After each interval take your pulse immediately, jot it down, and proceed as quickly as possible to the next interval. You can make up a chart like the one on page 61 or make photo copies if you like.

To take your pulse, you need only count for six seconds and then multiply by ten to estimate what the heart rate would be for a whole minute. Jot down just the six-second counts and do the arithmetic later.

These three heart rates at three well-defined workloads are your first reference points. After a week or two of your fitness program, repeat the reference workout at the same specific workloads (resistance settings and stroke rate) and again record your heart rate at the same three workloads. Over time, you should see a gradual decline in your rates for each workload. If not, you will have to work at a higher heart rate or increase the duration of your workouts.

By doing your reference workouts at the same time of day, on an empty stomach, and under cool conditions, you can be sure that your heart rate is related to your work capacity and not to other factors.

The heart rate needed to achieve a training effect varies greatly from individual to individual. You can get a rough estimate of your appropriate training heart rate by using a well-known formula that takes into consideration your age and what you feel is your current level of fitness:

Maximum Heart Rate $\times$ Intensity $=$ Training Threshold Heart Rate

Your maximum heart rate is estimated by subtracting your age from 220. The older you get the lower your maximum rate gets. Intensity refers to the percentage of your maximum heart rate you should try for. The intensity factor should be chosen according to your level of conditioning and general health factors. If you are already very fit, you might want to go for 85 percent of your maximum. But if you haven't done much more than run for the bus in the past few years, you'll gain cardiovascular benefits at an intensity of 65 percent of your maximum. In other words, if you are forty-five and sedentary, your equation would look like this: $(220 - 45) \times .65 = 114$. Or you may be somewhere in between. You can increase the intensity of exercise as your fitness increases.

ROW FOR YOUR LIFE
Reference Workout Chart

Date	Resting Heart Rate	Minutes of work	Strokes per Minute	Resistance Setting	Working Heart Rate	Minutes of work	Strokes per Minute	Resistance Setting	Working Heart Rate	Minutes of work	Strokes per Minute	Resistance Setting	Working Heart Rate
6/1	70	5	30	1	122	3	24	2	161	2	18	3	200
6/8	70	5	30	1	122	3	24	"	160	"	18	3	197
6/15	69	5	30	1	122	"	24	"	158	"	"	"	194
6/22	69	5	30	1	121	"	"	"	157	"	"	"	192
6/29	69	5	30	1	121	"	"	"	155	"	"	"	188
7/5	68	5	30	1	120	"	"	"	151	"	"	"	186
7/12	68	5	30	1	120	"	"	"	147	"	"	"	183
7/19	66	5	30	1	120	"	"	"	144	"	"	"	180

This example shows the progress of a young, fairly well conditioned subject over an eight-week period, under medical supervision. The Working Heart Rates that he achieved in the third phase of the reference workout were well above those indicated by the chart as the levels at which training could take place, and during the three-times-per-week exercise sessions he did not work at those elevated levels but at rates consistent with his age and condition as indicated by the Training Heart Rate Chart.

The quite low resistance setting on his machine did not move his heart rate into a training range in the first phase of his reference workout, and that makes this part of the reference workout a less sensitive barometer of conditioning than the next two. The higher resistance, that is, greater intensity of the second two phases yielded steady progress as indicated by a steady decline in his heart rate at a given load, of about 1.5 percent per week.

At some point in the program—different for each of us—progress stops as shown by the reference workouts. At that point, the intensity of the exercise needs to be increased in order to resume pushing down the heart rate at a given load. Alternatively, you can simply maintain your new level of fitness by keeping up with your program and checking your status from time to time to make sure you are not losing any ground.

ROW FOR YOUR LIFE
Reference Workout Chart

Late	Resting Heart Rate	Minutes of work	Strokes per Minute	Resistance Setting	Working Heart Rate	Minutes of work	Strokes per Minute	Resistance Setting	Working Heart Rate	Minutes of work	Strokes per Minute	Resistance Setting	Working Heart Rate

The resting heart rate can be used as another benchmark for the effectiveness of your training program. As your cardiovascular fitness improves, your resting heart rate should decrease. Before you begin your fitness program, establish your resting heart rate by checking it for three mornings before you get out of bed. Then check it at monthly intervals after you have begun training and whenever you plan to do a reference workout. If your resting heart rate does not decline after two or three months, reevaluate your program to determine if it is challenging your body. The resting heart rate, together with your reference workout for fitness tracking, should give you an indication of the value of your training.

How you feel during your exercise can also tell you if you are working hard enough. After a few minutes you should be breathing by mouth. If you can get sufficient oxygen breathing through your nose, you are not working hard enough. You should sweat, too. The sweat doesn't have to pour off of you, but you should feel flushed and a little damp. Sweating and mouth breathing are signs that you are challenging your body. And if you don't challenge your body, your body has no reason to change.

The accompanying chart indicates training heart rates for a range of ages and conditions, from quite sedentary at 60 percent of the maximum indicated rate to quite active at 85 percent. Training rates rarely exceed 85 percent, even in well-conditioned athletes.

It is important to bear in mind that the formula and the rates shown in this table are only guidelines. Use them to set an initial goal. After that, your reference workout will be the key indicator of the success of your own exercise program. There are so many individual variables in each of our bodies that the formula for estimating maximal heart rate, 220 minus age, can be off by plus or minus 12 beats per minute for two-thirds of the population.

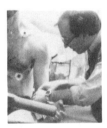

Checking Your Heart Rate

You can follow your pulse rate by checking it manually at your wrist or at the carotid arteries, which are found on both sides of the neck right below the jaw hinges. Or you may prefer to use a pulse monitor. An advantage of a pulse or heart-rate monitor is that it provides a continuous readout of the heart rate, without the need to stop exercising. Even a short pause in the course of exercise can result in a somewhat inaccurate heart-rate reading due to the rapid decrease in heart rate when activity is stopped.

Training Heart Rate Chart

AGE	CONDITION					
	FAIRLY SEDENTARY		FAIRLY ACTIVE		QUITE ACTIVE	
	60%	65%	70%	75%	80%	85%
18	121	131	141	152	162	172
22	119	129	139	149	158	168
26	116	126	136	146	155	165
30	114	124	133	143	152	162
34	112	121	130	140	149	158
38	109	118	127	137	146	155
42	107	116	125	134	142	151
46	104	113	122	131	139	148
50	102	111	119	128	136	145
54	100	108	116	125	133	141
58	97	105	113	122	130	138
62	95	103	111	119	126	134
66	92	100	108	116	123	131
70	90	98	105	113	120	128
74	88	95	102	110	117	124
78	85	92	99	107	114	121
82	83	90	97	104	110	117

Designing Your Program (Or Creating Your Own Exercise Equation)

All well-formulated fitness programs—whether employing running, swimming, rowing, or merely walking up and down the block—are built around combinations of intensity, duration, and frequency. Your needs and limitations will dictate what combination of these variables you utilize in designing your program.

Intensity—How Hard You Will Work—Intensity is the "sweat factor," and can be gauged by your heart rate. How hard you work within a given time frame (duration) is the key to successful conditioning. You will not experience a conditioning effect by exercising at a relatively low intensity unless you prolong the workout. For example, you can put your rower on a low-resistance setting and pull away leisurely. Fine, if you do this long enough for your heart rate to reach and pass your training threshold. Then again, you might be in a hurry. Pushing your heart rate into its training range by rowing faster or against greater resistance will do the job, too, and faster. But don't take that route until you have begun to get into shape.

Duration—How Long You Will Work—Duration and intensity are closely related in improving fitness, as explained above. What duration you choose will initially depend on your fitness level as well as your personal preference. Improvements in unfit individuals have been seen in sessions as short as five to ten minutes. High intensity workouts of ten to fifteen minutes can produce results in fit individuals. Some people prefer a longer workout—forty-five minutes to an hour or more.

Most people take the middle road. A long workout is boring and nonproductive. There are better things to do! A short, high-intensity workout can be painful and cause injuries and unnecessary fatigue. The twenty to thirty minute workout meets most needs and should be considered the minimum commitment by most people. This can be done at an intensity that is demanding but not exhausting. Of course, there are those with special needs who would be advised to go for a long, very low-intensity workout.

Frequency—How Often You Will Work—A once-a-week workout intense enough to keep your heart rate at your training level for twenty to thirty minutes will provide some cardiovascular improvement. Additional days, up to three or four per week, add to that improvement.

We recommend that you begin by plugging three days a week into your plan, with a resting day between. Exercising three days a week will allow you to gain noticeable cardiovascular benefits within two to six weeks. Your resting heart rate should decrease and your reference workout should also reveal some decrease in heart rate with the same amount of exercise. Whether you do your work on successive days or alternate days has no effect on conditioning as long as your heart rate is being raised to and kept in the training range for about 90 minutes per week for twenty to thirty minutes at a time. If you get tired, though, alternating days can be helpful because it will allow fatigued muscles to recover.

Later you can vary the frequency of the workout based on individual time constraints, how much you enjoy your exercise program, and how much other activity you get. By using your heart rate at identifiable workloads as a measure of progress, you can assure yourself that your training is effective at either increasing or maintaining fitness.

Frequency is an important consideration if you are combining dieting and exercise for weight control. Unless you greatly increase the intensity and duration of your workouts you will not burn as many calories on a three times a week schedule as you will on a five times a week schedule—or a seven-day-a-week schedule. For dieters, there are some real choices:

- On nonexercising days reduce intake by a few hundred calories.
- Exercise daily, and enjoy a few extra calories while losing weight.

Frequency is also an important consideration in gaining the psychological benefits of your exercise program and in increasing strength. With your rower, you can do some strength work on days when you are not scheduled for endurance training. Just set the load setting up a few notches, and row for five or ten minutes instead of twenty or thirty. Begin all workouts with a few minutes of warming up and stretching, and end them with a cool-down. In a very short time, you can give your body the opportunity to gain strength and flexibility, and your mind the benefits of physical activity.

Strength Exercises on Your Rower

Straightforward rowing, using the machines in the way they were most obviously designed to be used, is among the best of aerobic exercises, but some multi-purpose hydraulic machines lend themselves to alternate forms of exercise that you may wish to try for a change of pace or to strengthen specific muscle groups.

Our recommendations for the best aerobic effects are based on a high number of repetitions at a fairly low resistance setting. The following exercises, however, are intended to increase strength, which implies a different exercise equation. For these exercises, set the resistance into the middle to upper range on your machine and plan on doing a series of sets, a certain number of each exercise in turn in each set, repeating the full cycle several times.

Keep track of the settings you are using and the number of repetitions and cycles in each session. Start with a number of repetitions that is comfortable for you, and build from there. Your goal is to increase both resistance and the number of cycles you can perform. Build the number of repetitions of each exercise until you fill the time available. Then increase resistance, decrease the number of repetitions, and rebuild. Your heart rate during these exercises will not be a reliable indicator of your progress, but the increasing number of repetitions against higher levels of resistance will give you the good news.

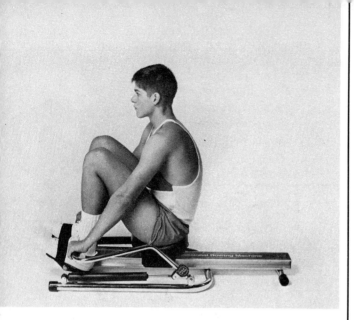

LEG PRESS

This exercise is actually a part of the rowing sequence that concentrates on the legs. Starting with the seat all the way forward and the arms straight, push with the legs until they are fully extended but not locked. Keep the arms and back straight.

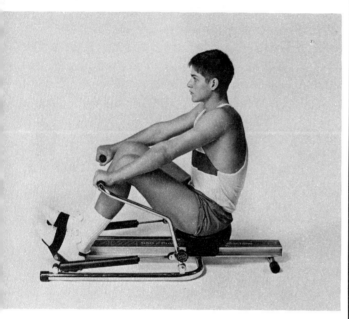

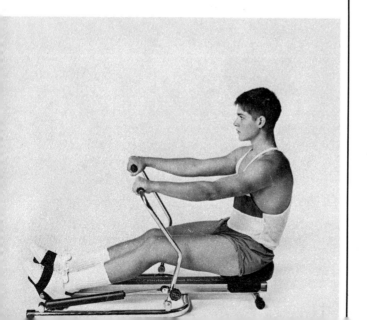

ARM PULLS

This exercise is good for the whole upper body, especially the arms. With the seat all the way back and your back held straight, alternate pulling each oar to your side. Keep your head up and try to keep the muscles of your neck and shoulders relaxed.

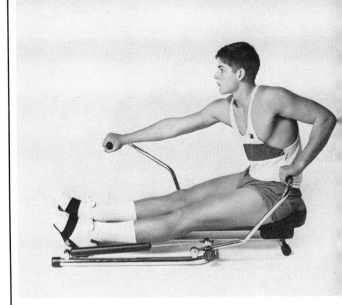

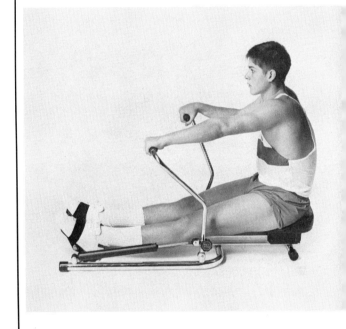

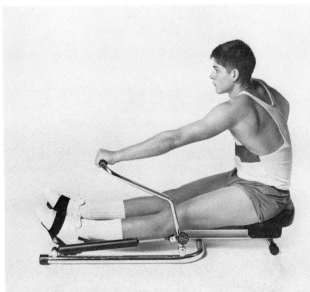

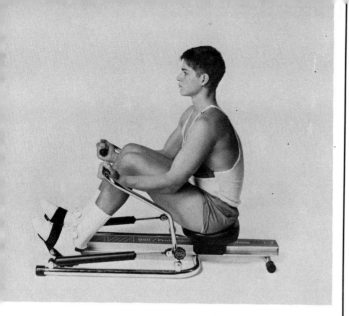

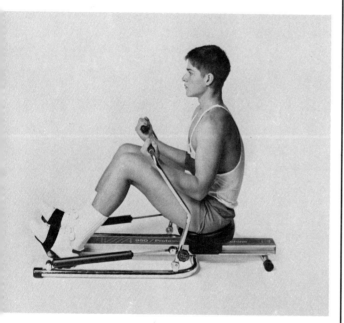

ARM CURLS

Curls are usually done with barbells, and are good for your forearms and biceps. The rower, with its variable setting, makes a good substitute. Move the seat forward until your elbows are approximately over the fulcrum of the oar. This setting will give you good leverage and minimize the strain on your lower back. If your rower seat can be locked in position, so much the better. With your grip reversed, i.e., with the palms facing up, lift against the resistance of the hydraulic pistons. Many hydraulic rowers are a little soft in the first few inches, and since arm curls require just that part of the stroke, you may want to set the resistance even higher for this exercise.

ARM PRESS

Arm presses are based on pushing, rather than pulling, so it is necessary to face backward with the rower seat held against the footplates (locked if possible) and your feet on the framework of the rower. Keeping your back straight, push with both hands until your arms are fully extended. Don't attempt to slide the seat forward and complete a full rowing stroke in reverse, but you may alternate arms as in the arm pull exercise.

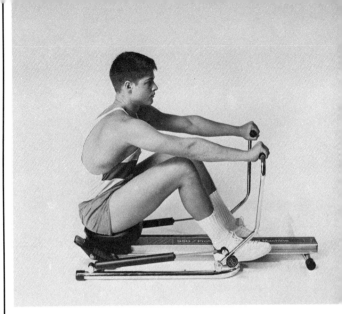

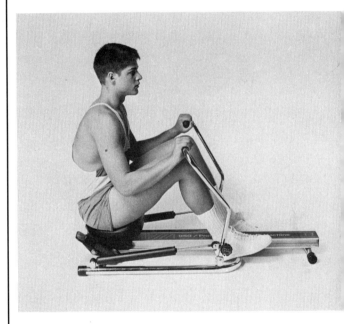

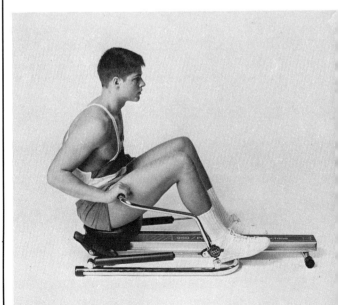

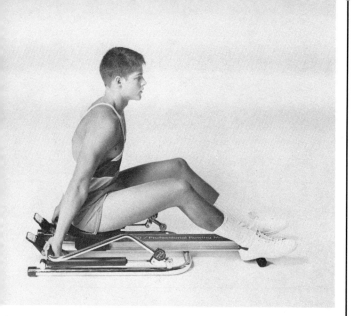

TRICEPS/DELTOID

The triceps make up the backs of your upper arms. They balance the work done by the biceps, but in the normal course of events do not get as much work and therefore have a tendency toward flabbiness. Still facing backward, with the seat locked (if possible) in a position that leaves your legs comfortably bent and your hands somewhat behind your back at the beginning of the cycle, lift the oars toward your armpits. As with the arm curls, this exercise may require a somewhat higher resistance setting in order to provide adequate work at the beginning of the hydraulic stroke.

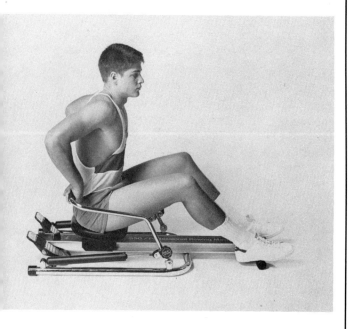

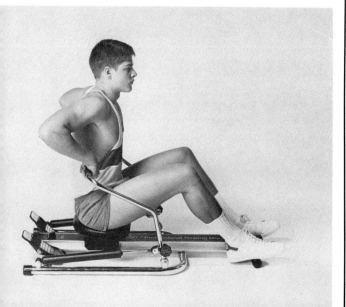

Maintaining Fitness

You may have been surprised at how quickly physiologic benefits can be gained through exercising no more than ninety minutes a week. A few short weeks really can bring about some remarkable changes. This is encouraging. But what is discouraging is that those benefits can vanish almost as quickly as they came. If you change your workout schedule from three times a week to once a week, half of your cardiovascular gains will be lost in ten weeks. Drop the program completely, and all the gains will be lost in about five weeks.

Maintaining conditioning requires a lifetime commitment to regular activity in the form of keeping your heart in a predetermined training range for approximately an hour and a half a week. It's not exactly the kind of commitment that forces you to give up your job and personal relationships, but it does take some determination. Planning an alternative exercise program for periods when you cannot carry out the rowing program you have set for yourself will be helpful. For instance, if business or vacation takes you away from your rower for a few weeks, plan some brisk half-hour walks, some swimming, or racquetball. Illness may interrupt your exercise schedule. When this happens, prepare for gradual resumption of your established program. Do not get discouraged if it takes two or three weeks to work your way back into a full program. Knowing that it is normal to have lost some capacity to exercise after inactivity will help you deal with this frustration.

Remember, what you are trying to do is set a pattern for lifetime fitness, not train for a marathon. Taking a few weeks to get up to, or back up to, a healthy level is okay.

Getting and Keeping the Exercise Habit

Once you have decided on the intensity, duration, and frequency at which you will work, give some thought to making the program as pleasant and convenient as possible. Making the program a real part of your life will depend on how you start out, when the workouts are scheduled, and what you do to avoid laziness and procrastination.

Plan to Ease into the Full Program—Let's say you've decided on 30 minutes on the rower at a heart rate of 75 percent of your maximum, three times a week. Fine. You may be able to do that from Day One—if you are already fit and if you have done some exercise using the upper body. Congratulations. Go to it.

Maybe you have been sedentary. Thirty minutes is a long time to sustain an unfamiliar activity. Pass up the soreness and fatigue and limit yourself to ten minutes or so a day for the first week or two, keeping the machine on a low-load setting. You will be amazed at how quickly and comfortably you can build to a full workout. With shorter initial workouts, you can pay some attention to technique and enjoy getting the feel of your machine.

As rowing becomes easier, add time, not resistance. Your first goal should be to complete the thirty minutes you have set for yourself, even if you must use a very light load throughout the program. When that thirty minutes is yours, add more resistance for part of the workout. But if you feel yourself getting ragged, back off. Lighten the load. At this point you will begin to monitor your heart rate more closely, either by use of a heart rate monitor or by simply pausing to check your pulse. Try to keep it in the range determined by the formula and your reference workout plus or minus five beats per minute.

Even if you are already in shape from another form of exercise, be prepared to find thirty minutes of rowing tough going at first. It might even be so hard that you will decide rowing and your body aren't compatible. Don't be hasty. There is a reason for the difficulty.

Your present state of cardiovascular fitness will make it easier for you to move into a full program than if you had been sedentary. But training is exercise-specific. All physiologic adjustments made in response to a specific exercise are not necessarily transferable to performance of another kind of exercise where different muscle groups are used. Your cardiovascular system reaps benefits, no matter what aerobic exercise you do, but using untrained muscle groups can put a load on your heart. For example, you may be able to jog at 85 percent of your maximum heart rate for thirty minutes very nicely. But try rowing at that maximum heart rate for thirty minutes and you will be in for a big surprise. It won't be easy. The same is true in going from rowing to jogging or to another sport. This is the reason rather active people can suffer heart attacks from the unfamiliar, but strenuous activity of shoveling snow.

Ease into your rowing program, gradually bringing these newly stressed muscle groups into play. Again, gradually work up to your intended duration and intensity so excessive fatigue doesn't spoil the joy of exercising.

Plan a Schedule You can Realistically Follow—Scheduling your workouts is like planning a diet. If you plan realistic calorie restrictions, you can stay with the diet. As a result, you will feel successful. This will reinforce your desire to slim down, and motivate you to cut out a few more calories. But suppose you suddenly decide on a 1000 calorie diet, with nothing but lean meat, a few complex carbohydrates, and some lettuce. You'll stray for sure. And feel like a failure. Before you know it, you'll be back on the chocolate chip and deep-fried track.

The same thing can happen with exercise. The plan must be realistic to be successful. Decide on a number of days that doesn't crowd your schedule. If you cannot realistically schedule three workouts, settle for two and call the third your "floating" workout. Fit it in whenever you can.

Then decide which days these will be—and when the workouts will be done. Choose a time that is usually yours, uninterrupted. Busy people don't have many such hours, but almost anyone can find three half hours a week. Take TV time. What about the 7 o'clock news? Or your favorite TV programs? Don't sacrifice them for rowing, merely combine rowing and TV. The beauty of the compact and quiet rowers is that you can work out in front of the TV, not bothering anyone by noise or clutter. Even the flywheel type machines are TV-compatible. Just turn the sound up a little and bring the TV to the machine.

Use your calendar as a reminder. Mark in your workouts for a month. When you cannot carry out a fully scheduled workout, block in a make-up session. Also, note the completion of floating workouts. Putting it down on paper and giving it the same importance as dentist appointments and party dates will help you treat the program as a serious commitment.

Plan for Lapses—If exercise were the first priority for most of us, you wouldn't be reading this book. Nor would we have written it. There wouldn't have to be people urging others on to exercise. Everyone would be running, biking, rowing, doing their own hard work, and walking instead of taking the bus. You just couldn't stop them.

But life isn't that way. Society is geared toward personal energy conservation rather than energy expenditure. Now you must nurture and develop attitudes that favor exercise and energy expenditure and regard them as investments in good health and good looks. Be prepared to allow several months for this attitude to bloom. In the meantime, sheer willpower and a few little tricks will have to suffice. No matter how carefully you have designed your program, there will be times—especially after the novelty wears off—when you will put aside workouts. Try some tricks to help you resist this urge.

On an exercise day, have your rower out and waiting for you when you get home from work. Put out your comfortable clothes, too.

Don't try to work in chores, phone calls, or a little reading before you exercise. Save them for later. You will have plenty of energy after your workout. Exercise will banish the fatigue of the workday, and you'll be able to accomplish a lot more work and fun on any evening that you exercise.

Promise yourself an abbreviated workout when you are tired. A half hour can seem like forever if you are tired, depressed, or rushed. Fifteen minutes may seem more appealing. Go for that instead. Chances are when that fifteen minutes has passed you will push on to complete the scheduled workout. The hardest part on a bad day is taking those first few pulls.

Keep an exercise diary with a partner. This will partially alleviate some of the loneliness of at-home exercise. Compare notes and progress and make plans to move to the next level of fitness together.

Your exercise diary need not be limited to entries about frequency, duration, and intensity—or even reference workouts. It could also include some information not expressed in numbers. What about that day when you noticed that your clothes fit you better, even though the scales said nothing about weight loss? Or the afternoon when you couldn't find a parking place within three blocks of the bank—and didn't care? Walking three blocks was exhilarating not exasperating. And the day you decided that you really did have time—and energy—to play some tennis or climb a mountain after work or on a weekend?

Such entries in your diary will tell you that your program is working to give you a better life and a better feeling about yourself right now. The longer term benefits of your personally designed exercise program will form the basis for many other entries in your fitness diary in the future.

Warming Up and Cooling Down

What does the warming up actually do? According to Dr. Frank G. Shellock, in the journal *Physician and Sportsmedicine,* the increase in body temperature and other changes brought about by a period of gradually more intense exercise has many important benefits. Warming up is just that—it warms up the body. A higher body temperature indicates that the system is prepared for the demands to be imposed upon it by activity.

The increase in body temperature stimulates the blood vessels to dilate, allowing increased blood flow to the muscles. This permits the necessary fuel and oxygen to be delivered to exercising muscles and limits the accumulation of metabolic by-products such as lactic acid. At a higher temperature, the hemoglobin releases oxygen more rapidly from red blood cells. These changes promote oxygen delivery to the muscles and cells and increase the body's ability to produce energy. The increased blood flow also helps to prevent injuries to muscles, tendons, ligaments, and other connective tissue. Muscle stiffness or flexibility in part depends on temperature, so cold muscles are more susceptible to damage than are warm muscles.

The mechanical efficiency of moving muscles is also improved at a higher body temperature. Muscular contraction is more rapid and forceful. The sensitivity of nerve receptors increases, as does the speed at which nervous impulses are transmitted.

The heart adapts to exercise better with a warm-up. Abnormal electrocardiographic changes unrelated to age or fitness have been observed in 70 percent of subjects who performed vigorous treadmill exercise for ten or fifteen minutes without a warm-up. However, these changes were not seen when these people performed the same exercise after a warm-up. This indicates that sudden, strenuous exercise can result in undesirable electrical activity by the heart.

The best way to warm up? Gradually raise the body temperature by activity such as calisthenics done with increasing intensity. Even better is to warm up by performing the exercise you plan to do—in this case rowing—at a very low intensity for several minutes, gradually working up to the intensity you desire. Then complete the warm-up by doing the stretching exercises shown on pp. 78–85 or other exercises that you may wish to do to stretch your muscles or increase your range of motion. This activity will increase your body temperature and allow you to rhythmically get into the workout.

Your body has two major pathways for generating energy: one requires oxygen and is called aerobic metabolism. The other can generate energy without oxygen, and is called anaerobic metabolism.

Aerobic metabolism generates most of the energy the body needs at rest or when the demand for power is low. As energy demand rises, however, oxygen-independent anaerobic metabolism gradually supplements the energy produced with oxygen. During strenuous exercise, the cardiovascular system cannot deliver enough oxygen to meet the muscles' demands. Anaerobic energy production compensates for the shortfall by generating more energy via the conversion of sugars. The end product of this process is lactic acid. When a large amount of energy is produced without oxygen, the accumulation of lactic acid (the familiar burning sensation) limits the duration of exercise. If such strenuous exercise is not followed by a proper cooling off period, muscle stiffness and even damage is more likely.

To avoid this condition, toward the end of your exercise session, gradually reduce the level of activity. Lighten the load and pull more slowly on the oars. Then, when you finish rowing, do some gentle stretching.

Another reason for cooling down is that the blood vessels have been dilated to accommodate a greater flow. An abrupt end to exercise may result in blood pooling in the legs, leaving an inadequate supply of blood for the brain. Fainting, arrythmias, or nausea can result.

Don't head for a hot shower immediately after strenuous exercise. Allow time for blood to be redistributed properly. The heat of a shower can cause blood vessels to dilate again to dissipate heat. Having both skin and muscle vessels open can result in a drop in blood pressure and fainting.

Avoiding Sore Muscles

Sore muscles cause many to drop out of fitness programs. Such muscle pain can be avoided by warming up and cooling down judiciously and by easing into the program gradually. While warmed up, it also helps to stretch for a few minutes before and after the workout. Stretching lengthens the muscles, increases blood flow to the areas being stretched, and increases range of motion. Stretching is also relaxing.

Stretching can present some hazard, however, if not done properly after warming up. Stretches should be gentle, reaching motions, with the extended position being held for several seconds. This allows time for the muscles and connective tissue to stretch out. Sudden, sharp movements, like quickly touching the toes, can pull and tear muscles. Refer to the warm-up section.

Avoiding Heat Stress

Once you are in the habit of exercising, you may hesitate to let heat change your schedule. Don't be rigid. The effects of heat can be insidious. Very often the real impact of overheating isn't apparent until the activity ceases.

In humans, body temperature is regulated in two general ways: physiologically and behaviorally. Under most conditions, the body's physiological mechanisms work quite well in coping with heat or cold, but they can be overwhelmed. This is where behavioral temperature regulation comes in. We use it everyday without thinking. Taking off and putting on clothes are examples, as are finding shade in hot weather and sunny spots in cool weather. Without thinking, in hot weather we change our behavior, doing less, eating lighter foods, and drinking more.

When environmental temperature falls, the body's 98.6° F core temperature is maintained by reducing blood to the extremities and by rerouting the blood flow. With the latter, the heat in arterial blood is transferred to venous blood before it can be lost. The temperature of the extremities can vary widely without harm. In extremely cold temperatures, however, there is a risk of ice crystal formation and punctured cells, known as frostbite.

In contrast to low temperatures, high temperatures can quickly disrupt metabolism. There are metabolic pathways in warm-blooded animals that do nothing except generate heat. A further increase occurs with exercise, as heat production accompanies energy production.

Sweating is the primary way humans dissipate the heat produced by the exercising muscles and the gut. As everyone knows from stepping out of a swimming pool on a breezy though warm day, evaporating water can make the body very cool. Over a half of a kilocalorie of heat is lost for every gram of water evaporated. There are 2 to 3 million sweat glands in a typical human. During exercise there is a ten-fold increase in blood flow to the skin. This brings heat from the deep tissues to the surface and promotes heat loss. The goal of body temperature regulation is to balance heat production with heat loss.

The most important route for heat loss is evaporation. How effectively heat is lost by sweating depends on how much water is evaporated. This, in turn, depends on the relative humidity and the maximum amount of water the air can hold. The colder the air, the less water it can hold. When the relative humidity is high, the capacity of air for additional water is limited, making it difficult for water to evaporate from the body. This is why humid days are so uncomfortable.

Sudden exposure to heat, particularly in combination with exercise, places an unusual strain on the cardiovascular system and can lead to stupor or fainting. This condition is called heat exhaustion, and is associated with low blood pressure, pale clammy skin, labored breathing, but normal body temperature. Lying down in a cool place is usually sufficient treatment, but if symptoms don't disappear quickly, i.e., in a few minutes, seek medical attention. The elderly are particularly intolerant of this kind of heat stress.

Heat stroke is a much more dangerous condition. It is associated with a hot, dry skin, a failure to sweat, and an elevated body temperature.

Unconsciousness, delirium, and serious brain and nerve damage can occur. People over sixty-five are particularly susceptible.

Use common sense during indoor as well as outdoor exercise on hot days. Consider the humidity as well as the actual temperature. A temperature of 86°F (30°C) and a relative humidity near 100 percent is as dangerous as 95°F (35°C) and a low humidity. If you want to work out and the temperature and the humidity are high, cut the time in half and lower the intensity. You will still keep your muscles in play and experience the fresh feeling of having done some physical work, but you will not expose yourself to the dangers of overheating.

When the weather turns hot, allow yourself time to get used to the heat. Heat tolerance can build by increasing the capacity to sweat, but this increased tolerance wears off within a few weeks.

In hot weather you will lose fluids constantly even though you may not seem to be sweating much. This means that you must increase your fluid intake beyond what you might feel like drinking. Drink plenty of water before and after your workout. Then drink frequently throughout the day. You will know that your fluid intake is adequate if your urine is pale rather than a deep yellow. Don't take salt pills unless advised to by your physician. The salt you get in your food should be sufficient unless you are working in a hot environment, which can lead to a large amount of salt being lost in sweat.

Warm-up and Stretching Exercises

Warm-up and cool-down routines are important to an overall fitness program. They prepare your muscles for demands of work or exercise, and they help to clear the accumulated wastes from them after the workout is finished. Warm-up and stretching can help prevent strains and other injuries, while the cooldown phase will head off post-exercise soreness.

With a rower, the warm-up and cool-down can take place on the machine itself, simply by working slowly with five or ten minutes of low resistance, low stroke-rate rowing at the beginning and end of the training effect workout.

Stretching exercises are also important, and elite athletes like Barbara Kirch will typically spend five or ten minutes warming up on the rower and then go through a stretching routine like the one shown here.

Remember, these are not calisthenic exercises in which you are using weight and momentum to provide some of the stretch—which can shock or damage tissue. These are done slowly and are merely intended to stretch already warmed up muscles to prepare them for the more vigorous work that will follow. Do each one for a slow five-count.

By the way, these stretching exercises are fine to do even when you do not intend to follow through with a hard workout.

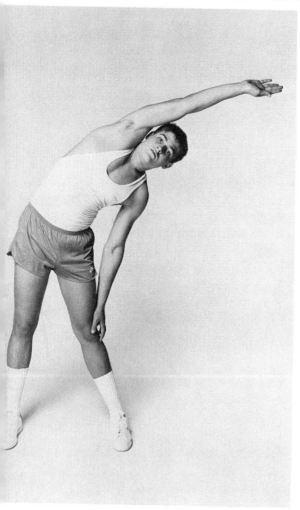

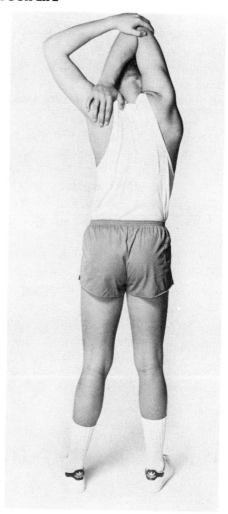

1. Start with your feet spread a bit farther apart than the width of your shoulders. Raise one arm over your head and lean to the opposite side, keeping your legs straight. You should feel a gentle tug along the side of your ribs and waist. Repeat to the other side.

2. With your feet in the same stance and your body straight, pull one arm up behind your head until the elbow points straight up. Use your other hand to pull your elbow toward the center line of your back. Repeat with the other arm.

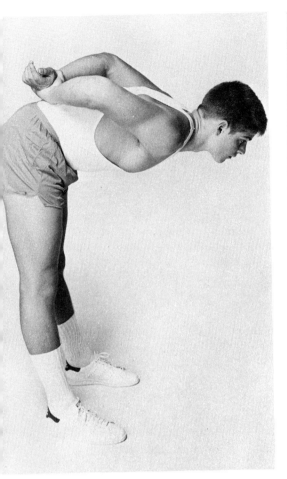

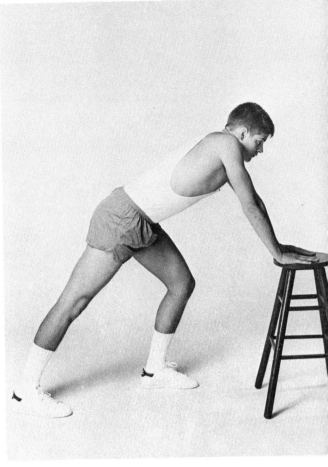

3. With your feet together and legs straight, clasp your hands behind your back and bend forward to stretch the backs of your thighs. There is no special virtue in touching your toes, and trying for them can put an unnecessary strain on your lower back. Keeping your hands behind you has the effect of focusing your attention on your hamstrings while reducing some of the load on your back.

4. With one foot forward and the other leg straight, lean against any handy wall or object. Lean as far forward as you can while keeping both feet flat on the floor. Repeat with the other leg back. This one is a favorite of joggers, whom you often see trying to push over trees and fences in the park. It stretches the calf muscles.

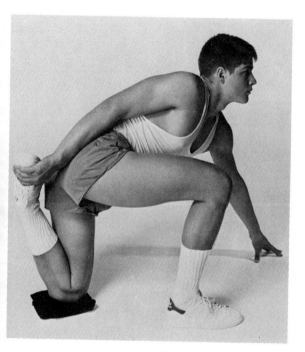

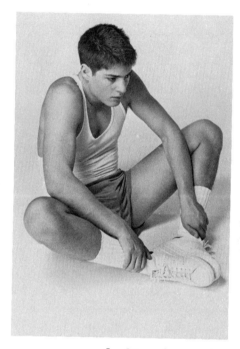

5. This one could be called a sprinter's stance. Your weight is on one knee, which you will want to pad a little. The other leg is forward for balance. With the hand opposite the load-bearing knee, grasp that foot and pull it up tight against your buttocks. Repeat with the other leg. Be careful with this stretch if you have chondromalacia—deterioration of the cartilage behind the knee found in many runners—or other knee problems.

6. Sit and press the bottoms of your feet flat against each other. With your hands on your feet, press outward against the insides of your legs with your elbows. This exercise stretches the groin muscles.

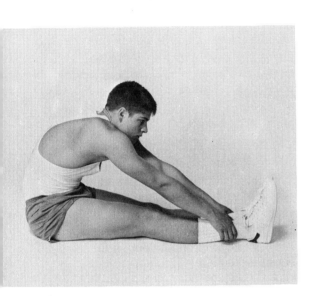

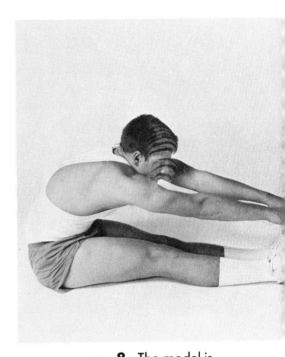

7. Sit, lean forward, and grasp your shins, being sure to bend from the waist and not the shoulders or upper back. The idea is to bring your stomach closer to your thighs, not your nose to your knees. This is similar to the bending over from the waist exercise but more controlled. Don't overdo it.

8. The model is showing off here. A young, superbly conditioned athlete has this kind of flexibility, but he may also have somewhat longer-than-usual arms, or shorter legs. Most of us cannot do this and should not try, but if you are naturally flexible in this position, by all means use this stretch.

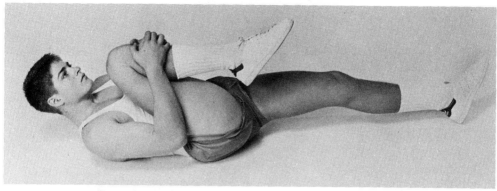

9. Lying on your back, pull one knee up toward your chest. Raise your head and shoulders off the mat, so that your forehead can just touch your knee. Repeat with the other leg. This stretches the lower back and buttocks.

10. Still on your back, raise one leg at a time, keeping the knee straight. Grasp your shin as far up as you can and pull toward your chest. This exercise is similar to toe touching but more controlled. Be careful. If you have trouble keeping your knees straight, or feel a strain on your lower back, bend the knee that is still on the floor. Repeat with the opposite leg.

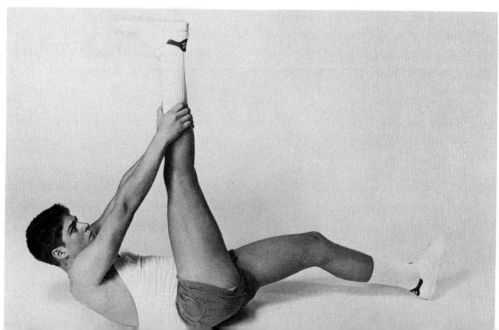

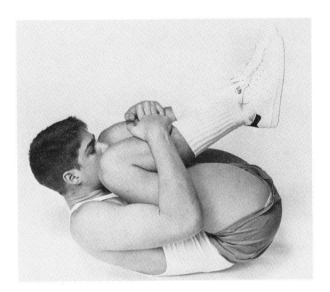

11. Pull both legs up toward your chest and tuck your head toward your knees, just like a mighty cannonball into the swimming pool.

12. Sitting up now, cross one leg over the other and pull the top knee up toward your chest, crossing both arms over it. Pull in gently. Repeat with the other leg. This is another buttocks stretch.

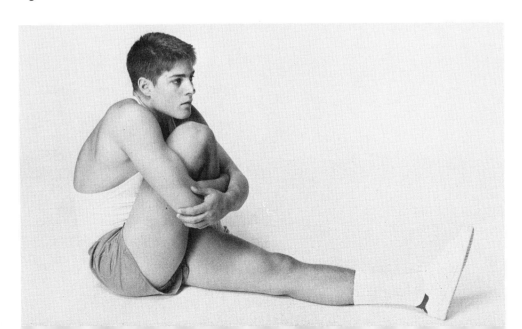

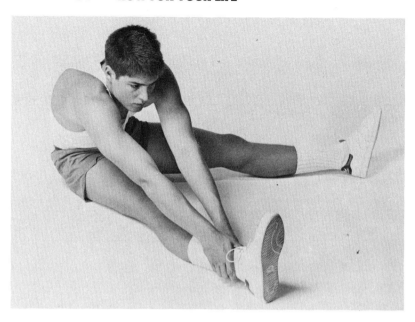

13. Sitting up with your legs spread out, grasp one shin and bend your head toward that knee, being careful of your lower back and hamstrings. Repeat with the other leg.

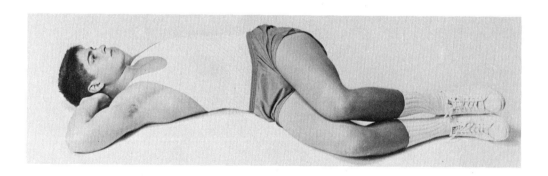

14. With your hands clasped behind your head and your elbows and shoulders touching the mat, keep your knees together and turn your hips so that your right knee comes as close as possible to the mat. Repeat by turning to the left.

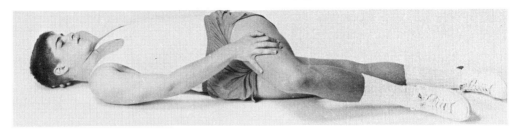

15. With your shoulders still flat to the mat and your left hand still behind your head, cross your left knee over the extended right leg and use your right hand to press that knee down toward the mat. Repeat to the other side.

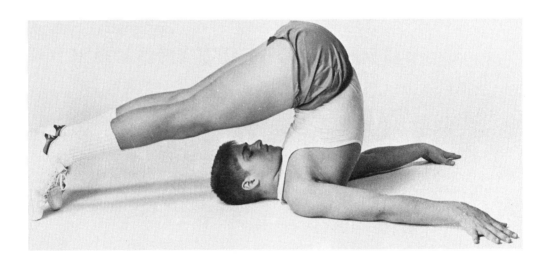

16. Head and shoulders flat to the mat, arms extended for balance, raise both legs up and over so that your toes touch the mat behind you, being careful of your lower back, as always.

6

Nutrition: Fuel for the Fire

The human body is indirectly powered by the sun. The sun bombards the earth with packets of energy called photons. Plants trap this energy, usually with the help of a green crystal-like pigment called chlorophyll, and use it primarily to organize carbon (C) from the carbon dioxide (CO_2) in the air, hydrogen (H) from water (H_2O), and nitrogen (N) from the soil or air, into various chemical combinations, including fats, carbohydrates, and proteins. The nutrients animals need to survive can be obtained directly from plants, or indirectly by eating the meat of plant-eating animals. Without the sun's energy there would be no foundation for the sometimes lengthy food chain we all depend on.

Food is broken down into its component parts by the digestive system and transported to the various cells for storage or for use. Depending on prevailing needs, your body's chemical machinery (metabolism) might gradually release the energy trapped within carbohydrates or fats to perform work, or use the protein subunits called amino acids to build or repair tissues. Without a constant flow of building blocks and energy, the body's high level of organization cannot be maintained and death occurs.

Practical Dietary Guidelines

False information and fads mislead many who are trying to maintain a balanced and adequate diet. We will provide you with simple and concise information along with guidelines for developing a sensible approach to eating.

The trend over the last century has been toward eating less of grains, vegetables, roughage, complex carbohydrates, and more of refined sugar, animal protein, and snack foods. Fortunately, there is evidence that this trend is reversing. The number of "health foods" available, even on the supermarket shelves, attests to this. Eating nutritionally sound meals does not mean limiting yourself to specially prepared health foods, however.

Except for price, health foods are usually no different from any other grocery store food. Plants take up only inorganic nutrients; therefore it doesn't matter if they are fertilized with organic or synthesized fertilizers.

A key to improving athletic performance or increasing the capacity for prolonged heavy labor is often a simple matter of eating enough food, primarily in the form of carbohydrates, to meet the increased caloric demand. Athletes who are actively training and competing often consume inadequate kilocalories (Kcal, sometimes referred to as calories) in relation to their energy output. The resulting weight loss and impaired performance can be avoided by eating frequent small meals high in complex carbohydrates throughout the day.

Athletes, knowing the value of carbohydrates, often limit their intake of fat and protein and consume 60–70 percent or more of their calories as carbohydrates. This habit is not necessarily bad if the diet falls within the broad guidelines of proper nutrition. Diets unusually restricted in fat and protein content, however, have been associated with heart attacks in highly trained long-distance runners. It is important for everyone, including elite athletes, to eat a varied and balanced diet that contains an adequate number of calories. The middle ground, where carbohydrates constitute 65 percent of the total caloric intake, is a sensible course.

Can Vegetarians Be Successful Athletes?

There are different types of vegetarians: lacto-ovo vegetarians, who eat both dairy products and eggs, in addition to vegetables and grains; lactovegetarians, who add only dairy products; and pure vegetarians, who eat no animal products at all. Many talented athletes, including several elite rowers, have had very successful careers on vegetarian diets, but you should consult a physician or highly qualified nutritionist before embarking on a vegetarian diet. Pure vegetarians, particularly those with a high energy expenditure, can have potentially serious problems with malnutrition.

Maintaining an Energy Balance

The goal of a balanced diet is to have caloric INPUT = OUTPUT. When food intake decreases below approximately 1800 Kcal per day, the amount of work that can be done decreases. For example, the work output of German steel workers and coal miners during World War II decreased in parallel with the declining calorie content of their food.

Active people should not generally need vitamin or mineral supplements, but they do require a greater caloric intake to meet their increased energy output, and additional water to control body temperature and meet metabolic needs. Whether vitamin supplements can increase the performance of elite athletes remains to be seen and deserves research.

A proper nutritional balance can be difficult to achieve in sedentary individuals. When caloric intake is adjusted to caloric output, there is the risk of an inadequate vitamin/mineral intake. Either vitamin and mineral supplements can be taken, or a more active lifestyle can be pursued. The more you do, the more you can eat without experiencing a weight gain. In addition, if you are eating a balanced diet, you will consume an adequate amount of the various vitamins and minerals.

Carbohydrates

Carbohydrates are easily metabolized and are very important in keeping the metabolic fire going. For a normal adult, carbohydrates should make up approximately 65 percent of the calories consumed, preferably in the form of complex carbohydrates—grains, cereals, vegetables, potatoes, rice, etc. Although carbohydrates constitute only 1–2 percent of the body's total energy stores, they serve a number of important functions. Without carbohydrates, for example, red blood cells, nerve cells, and the kidneys cannot function normally. In addition, carbohydrates permit high energy output during exercise by serving as the fuel for glycolysis, a metabolic pathway that produces energy without oxygen.

During strenuous exercise, energy is generated without oxygen by converting glucose into lactic acid. The liver, through the glucose–lactic-acid cycle, uses the energy in fat to convert lactic acid back to glucose. This process conserves the body's limited carbohydrate stores, reduces the need to form glucose from protein, and makes it possible for skeletal muscles to produce large amounts of energy.

Eating sugar or simple carbohydrates immediately before or during exercise can interfere with the regulation of blood sugar levels. When foods high in simple carbohydrates are consumed, blood sugar levels rise. This increase in blood sugar, however, is only temporary. The body responds by increasing the concentration in the blood of the sugar storage hormone, insulin. This often results in a "rebound" decrease in blood sugar to a very low level.

Fat

Fat has the highest caloric content per weight of any fuel source. Ideally, fat should make up only 20–30 percent of the total dietary Kcals. A simple way to reduce the number of calories in a diet, and avoid a high level of fat in the blood, is to eat a low-fat, low-cholesterol, high fiber, high carbohydrate diet. Eating an excessive amount of food from any source, however, can result in high fat levels in the blood.

Using unsaturated fats rather than saturated fats is thought to prevent clogging of the vessels that supply blood to the heart muscle. Dietary cholesterol and saturated fat intake can be reduced by eating:

- more fish or skinless turkey or chicken; less red meat;
- more vegetable oil or margarine; less butter, bacon fat, coconut oil, and palm oil;
- more low-fat, skim milk cheeses; less Cheddar, Swiss, and cream cheese;
- fewer egg yolks.

Protein

Protein, made up of subunits called amino acids, should constitute 10–15 percent of the calories in a diet. This will provide sufficient amino acids to build and repair tissues. Protein can be obtained either by eating meat, which contains all the essential amino acids, or by eating foods which have complementary combinations of essential amino acids. For example, corn and beans eaten together provide all of the necessary essential amino acids. Obtaining essential amino acids from plant or dairy sources can help reduce the fat content in your diet because meat, particularly red meat, can be high in saturated fat.

The human body does not store protein. When protein is eaten in excess of bodily needs, it ends up being used as an expensive fuel. Protein is also a less than ideal source of immediate energy. The breakdown of protein produces nitrogen containing waste products such as ammonia which then have to be detoxified and excreted.

Is there an increased protein need with exercise? If you are eating a balanced diet, the increase in food consumed in response to activity will be accompanied by an increase in the amount of protein eaten, which should meet any extra needs. Young athletes who are still growing, or those who are training for strength and seek to increase their muscle mass, may benefit from an increased protein intake.

Fiber

Fiber, also referred to as roughage, is primarily made up of the nondigestible cellulose part of plants, and serves to increase the bulk of foodstuffs. Since high-fiber food takes longer to chew and swallow, it is often gratifying to eat, and results in a feeling of satisfaction. In contrast, the large amount of energy per weight in highly refined foods makes it easy to consume many calories in a short time and still feel unsatisfied. Because dietary fiber is indigestible, it increases the size of stools and speeds their movement through the digestive tract. Generally, processed food has a low fiber content, whereas unprocessed food generally has a higher fiber content. Dietary fiber may play a role in reducing the incidence of colon cancer. The importance of fiber in the management of diabetes is currently under investigation.

Water

A lean human being is around 75 percent water. All the chemical reactions within the body take place in water and water is important in transporting and disposing of waste products.

How often and how much one urinates, along with the color of the urine, are good indicators of hydration. If your urine is dark, it may indicate a need to increase water intake. When an individual is drinking too little water, the body compensates not only by making more concentrated urine, but by removing more of the water from the feces residing in the large bowel, increasing the risk of constipation.

It takes water to digest, process, and store food. A large amount of water is associated with stored carbohydrates, for example. The rapid initial weight loss at the beginning of a diet is due to the loss of carbohydrates and their associated water, rather than of fats.

Vitamins and Minerals

Vitamins and minerals are not used for energy or as building blocks, but are needed in minute quantities for normal metabolism. Is it necessary to take vitamin and mineral supplements? For the typical person eating an adequate and balanced diet, probably not. Additional iron and folic acid, however, are needed during pregnancy when the fetus is growing rapidly. After pregnancy, iron stores are sometimes lowered and extra iron is advisable. Anemia is also a common problem in menstruating women. Iron supplements can help to alleviate this problem

Most vitamins are water soluble and any excess is readily excreted. The vitamins A, D, E, and K, however, are fat soluble and can accumulate in body fat to a point where they can cause a toxic reaction. These vitamins can be remembered by the mnemonic, ADEK, which suggests ADDICT. Excessive amounts of certain trace elements can also be toxic.

Salt (sodium chloride) is a necessary micronutrient and iodized salt is a convenient way to avoid goiter formation. The typical western consumption of salt far exceeds need, and can even lead to high blood pressure or hypertension. One reason it is difficult to keep track of salt intake is that many processed foods are high in salt. It may be wise to limit the use of salt in home cooking or as a table condiment. In contrast, salt lost through sweating during work in hot conditions can lead to an increase in the need for dietary salt, but consult your physician before taking salt tablets.

Food Allergies

Food allergies, particularly lactose intolerance, and hence, intolerance of milk and dairy products, are more and more common. The increasing variety of foods and additives we are exposed to contributes to this trend. Food allergies have many expressions including upset stomach, poor digestion, asthma, headache, and fatigue. If you suspect you have food allergies, *Basics of Food Allergy* by J.C. Breneman (Charles C. Thomas, 1984), is a good source of additional information.

7

Advice and Program for Older Exercisers

Physical Activity—A Means to a Healthier and More Productive Maturity

As a nation, we are growing older. Half the population is now older than fifty. One thousand persons become sixty-five every day and join the age group that traditionally has been considered elderly. A nation can benefit greatly from the experience and stability of a mature population. Whether this will be true for the United States in the closing years of the twentieth century will depend on the physical condition of the older segment of the population.

There is no doubt that with age the human body changes. And usually not for the better. The external changes—graying, balding, wrinkling—are obvious. Within the body, changes are taking place, too, and these are the ones that lead to the physical degeneration that ends in chronic illness and disability. But there is good news, too. Scientific evidence indicates that this inevitable winding down of the human machine does not have to take place at the rate we so frequently witness. Regular, fairly vigorous activity can stave off the effects of aging and prolong our productive years.

To describe how important activity is to people in all age groups, including those in late-middle and old age, it is necessary to provide some background information on the changes that have been observed with age. Then we can tell you how activity has been shown to lessen these changes.

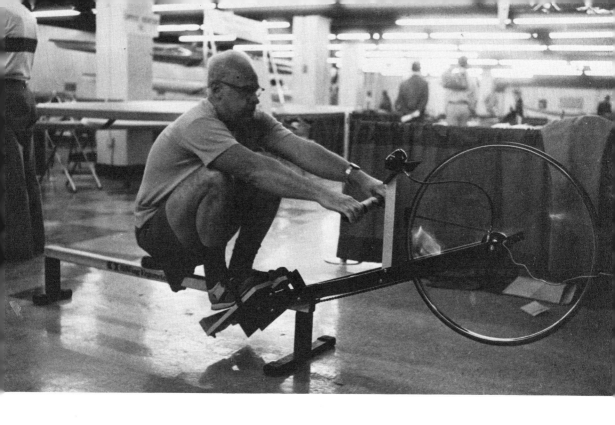

An *older exerciser working out on the Concept II at a Philadelphia "erg race."*

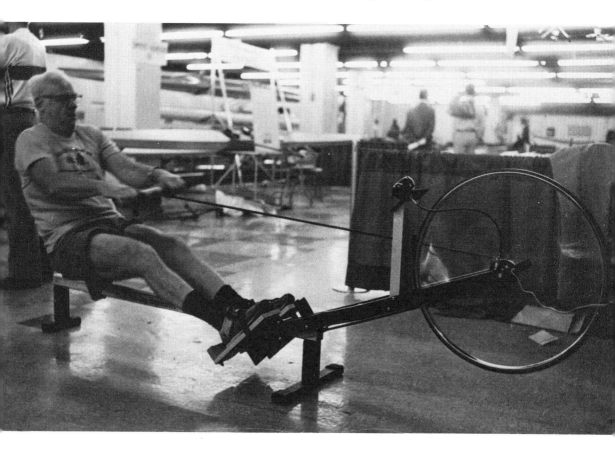

The Effects of Age

The functional capacity of most organ systems declines at a rate of 0.75 to 1 percent per year from their peak at around the age of thirty. Strength and muscle mass decline at the same rate, as do cardiac output, maximal oxygen consumption, heart rate, and the capacity of the respiratory system. The respiratory and circulatory systems of older people adapt more slowly than those of younger people when muscular work is done. The production of most hormones is reduced and there is a tendency toward atherosclerosis.

By age seventy, women have lost 30 percent of their bone mass; males have lost 15 percent. This loss begins in women by about ages thirty to thirty-five and in men from fifty to fifty-five. Bone strength is thereby decreased and there is increased risk of fracture. Joint flexibility is reduced 25 to 30 percent. Joints stiffen and range of motion decreases. Among the causes are wear and tear and thickening of the joint capsule. The chest stiffens, making it harder to move air in and out of the lungs.

In one study of 65-year-old subjects, the difference in muscle strength between subjects varied from 54 to 65 percent of that of 25-year-olds. This loss of muscle strength can be attributed to loss of muscle mass. Coordination also diminishes.

It's Not Just the Calendar

Is this degree of deterioration inevitable? Many say not. Scientists now think that 50 percent of this diminished function can be attributed to disuse and can be prevented by physical activity. They also feel that some functions can be restored by activity.

Biological and chronological age are not always in tandem, and the greater the age, the greater the variation between individuals. An active lifestyle seems to have a bearing on the aging process, as, of course, does heredity and personal health history.

The ability to do hard work doesn't just shut off at a certain birthday. Older persons working side by side at active occupations very often do the same job with the same intensity as their younger co-workers. In a study of work in men approaching sixty-five, it was found that strength and endurance on the job did not differ from that of men as young as twenty-two who were engaged in the same work.

Usually, physiological alterations such as a reduction in maximal oxygen consumption and a smaller stroke volume with exercise occur in the absence of heart disease. For this reason—and because research shows that some of the decline can be reversed or even prevented by exercise training—inactivity no doubt contributes to much of the decline in the first place. In athletes, the maximal oxygen consumption declines with age at the same rate as for sedentary individuals. But because athletes have a higher level in early adulthood, their maximal oxygen consumption, even though declining, will be high compared with those less active individuals of the same chronological age. An example of this was a 65-year-old athlete with a maximal oxygen consumption approximately the same as that of a sedentary 25-year-old.

Staying in shape has an effect on mental capacity, too. Cognitive function appears to be improved in older people who participate in a sport, as compared to those who are unfit. Several studies point out that the functional capacity of the cardiovascular system is a factor in reducing problems with short term memory in the elderly. There is also a relationship between the cardiovascular system and the ability to react to stimuli. Middle-aged and elderly sportsmen have shorter reaction times than their more sedentary contemporaries.

An active lifestyle in older people may even prolong life. Death rates have been found to be related to activity. In men aged sixty to sixty-four there were 4.9 deaths per 100 in those taking no exercise and 0.92 in those taking regular heavy exercise. The positive effect of exercise increased further with age. In men aged sixty-five to sixty-nine, the death rates in inactive persons was 10.33/100 vs. only 1.38/100 among the exercisers.

Another survey showed that older men who performed regular physical training through many years had significantly lower serum cholesterol levels than did an inactive control group. Because high serum cholesterol levels are associated with cardiovascular disease, it can be postulated that these men should expect increased longevity.

The Response of the Mature Body to Conditioning

But what about you? If you are over fifty and have not had an active occupation, participated in a strenuous sport, or exercised regularly, can you still slow or reverse the insidious effects of aging? Ideally, the habit of regular training should be established early in life. However, exercise in older people, even if they have been sedentary, can reverse some already existing effects of aging—or of a sedentary existence. You can live vigorously until your time is up instead of giving in to decline in middle age.

What has emerged from research on men and women well into their seventies is that the relative effect of training in older people is comparable to that in younger people. For example, in men fifty to sixty-three years of age, the improvement in maximal oxygen consumption (19 percent) was the same as their counterparts who ranged in age from thirty-four to fifty. This improvement was accomplished in just ten weeks of aerobic training. An exercise program for women from fifty-two to seventy-nine-years-old resulted in a 37 percent improvement in physical work capacity and a 20.8 percent increase in maximal oxygen consumption. Other research studies of training in the elderly have shown increases in maximal oxygen consumption, stroke volume, and cardiac output that make up for half the 30 percent decrement due to age.

These statistical changes can be translated into everyday advantages. An increased aerobic capacity simply means that activities that require exertion will be easier. Tasks like taking care of the yard, carrying packages from the store to the car, and washing windows can be done without fatigue. The depression that comes from finding routine tasks difficult can be avoided. Travel and hobbies can be enjoyed without worry. Being in good physical condition can mean the difference between enjoying pleasures for their own sake or simply treating them as obstacle courses.

Increase of bone mass has been reported after a program of physical exercise. Bone mineralization improves, probably from improved circulation and increased gravitational and muscular stress that influence the cellular activity of the bones. This is an important factor in lessening the chances of fractures.

Many previously vigorous older people can trace the decline of their health to a broken bone or an illness which required either bed rest or inactivity. Bed rest, even if only for a few days or a week or two, can result in a drastic loss of aerobic capacity in older people. This loss of cardiovascular fitness results in dropping out of activities which had been routine prior to the fracture, thus setting off a vicious cycle of further decreased function, decreased activity, and mental depression. Such a downward spiral of function can be avoided, if an injury or illness occurs, by recognizing its dangers and gradually working back into a more active life.

Exercise in elderly people can also strengthen muscles. Because the size of the muscles does not increase, the increase in strength is thought to be due to increased neural activitation and better oxygen delivery to the muscles. Joints also become more flexible. The more joints involved in the activity, the better. This is one reason to recommend calisthenics or stretching exercises that put multiple joints through their range of motion before beginning your aerobic program.

Physical stimulation keeps the endocrine glands from atrophying, thereby becoming less responsive. Failure to keep the endocrine system ready and able to react to stress is one of the main reasons older people cannot function effectively. The mild stress of exercise can tune up the adrenal system so that a person can successfully cope with both the daily and the severe stresses of life.

The fact that older people who exercise regularly feel better should not be lost in all of these facts and statistics. Even if cardiac function were not improved, possibly leading to a longer life, or muscles were not strengthened, allowing for a wider range of activities, exercise would still pay off. Older persons who exercise are less concerned about their health, sleep better, have a better self-image and are more sociable. Flexible joints and responsive muscles allow them to enjoy many activities for which there is now time. An improvement in coordination and reaction time can result in improvements in both confidence and safety.

Exercise can break the vicious cycle of inactivity, indifference and weakened functioning that comes from sedentary living as well as aging, and can enable people of all ages to look forward to each day with enthusiasm.

Practical Advice

Specialists in aging very often divide older people into two groups: the young—old, from age fifty-five to seventy-five; and the old—old, who are over seventy-five. But, of course, chronological age does not tell the whole story. Approximately 50 percent of the decline in function seen in the older population as a whole is due to disuse rather than to aging itself. Regular exercise can retard this process or, if it has already taken place, partially reverse it. But in designing an exercise program for older people, certain things should be kept in mind.

One of these is the type of exercise. Most therapists recommend active rhythmic use of large muscle groups and avoidance of stress on the joints. The program should aim to improve joint flexibility, muscle tone, and cardiorespiratory endurance. Highly competitive activities that involve sudden bursts of effort should be avoided.

Rowing, of course, meets these criteria either as a single form of exercise or a back-up for other means of fitness. Walking, dancing, and cycling are also excellent forms of exercise for everyone. Older people who enjoy them should continue on with them.

But this isn't always possible. Orthopedic problems sometimes prohibit dancing or walking, if only temporarily. The weather can be the deciding factor for cycling or other outdoor activities. A partner might not always be available for activities such as dancing or sports like tennis. Very often it is just such situations—weather, illness, or unavailability of companions—that get older people out of the exercise habit. Many never go back to the activity—or when they try to go back they find that they have become out of shape and easily fatigued. Fatigue cuts down on the pleasure. Discouraged, they give up and pursue sedentary pleasures.

Having a rower at home and getting used to using it a few times a week can be an excellent safeguard against the time when the recreation you like is not available. Through rowing you can maintain strength and stamina so that when the time is right you can return to the activities you most enjoy.

Rowing uses the major muscle groups of both upper and lower body. Moderate rhythmic exercise using these large muscles is associated with less of a rise in blood pressure and less work for the heart than similar work done using small muscle groups, such as those in the forearm or hands, or with the use of small weights or squeeze gadgets. There is also less load on the heart when large muscle groups are used rhythmically. Isometric exercises, such as pushing against resistance or lifting weights, cause a sudden rise in the blood pressure and may lead to circulatory failure.

An exercise program for older people, as with everyone, should be designed around intensity, duration, and frequency. Age, however, will play a part in deciding the exact program to undertake. And, of course, a preprogram physical examination should not be omitted.

Intensity—Begin by inserting your age into the formula: (220 − age) × intensity = training threshold. See the table on page 63.

The intensity recommended for younger people ranges from 65 to 85 percent. There is some disagreement as to what intensity (heart rate) will provide a training effect in older people, although it is agreed upon that a lower range is desirable. Most commonly, the range recommended is from 40 to 70 percent of maximal heart rate. However, exercising at a heart rate of 30 to 40 percent of the maximum (220 − age) has produced improvements in maximal oxygen consumption comparable to that in persons exercising at a 60 to 75 percent intensity. Decide upon a reasonable range for you with your doctor. Consider your current state of conditioning as well as your general health. If you have been inactive, start at a lower level and work up. You can determine if you are experiencing a conditioning effect by checking your heart rate at specific workloads in a reference workout. See page 62.

Duration—Thirty to sixty minute sessions, including a warm-up and cool down, are generally recommended. At a lower intensity level, it is necessary to increase the duration to achieve a training effect. Don't aim for the whole thirty minutes—let alone an hour—right away. Instead, ease into the program, letting your muscles get used to this new form of exercise. Even a fifteen- to twenty-minute workout will provide results. To gain strength on the rower and build up endurance, do two workouts a day, for example—two fifteen-minute periods or even two thirty-minute periods. As you begin to work up to the intensity appropriate for you, drop one of the workouts. Don't be impatient. It may take several weeks before you can comfortably complete a full workout.

Frequency

Working out regularly, at least every other day, is important for older people. No more than two days should separate each session. Regularity keeps the muscles and joints in good order and maintains flexibility and muscle tone. Regular daily activity is important for older people, especially those who are retired and live in areas where the weather prevents year 'round outdoor activity. A good idea might be to use the rower at the appropriate intensity for cardiac fitness for three days a week, then on the other days pay attention to the musculoskeletal system. Go through the warming up and cooling down routine, doing stretches and calisthenics that will keep the joints limber and muscles supple. Also, for strength, use the rower for five or ten minutes on a heavier than usual load.

Warming Up and Cooling Down

Because the body becomes less supple with age, activity that focuses on maintaining a wide range of motion should be done often. The principles of the warm-up and cool-down are the same for everyone. However, in older people the warm-up should be extended both from the cardiovascular and musculoskeletal standpoint. It should include some gentle warming up, then stretching through the full range of motion of joints. To avoid soreness and injury, don't repeat any one motion or exercise more than three or four times. Also, include some low-intensity rowing in your warm-up, gradually working yourself into a rhythmic motion. Because the heart rate returns to normal less quickly in the elderly, there should be a longer cooling down period.

Heat Stress

A decreased capacity to sweat comes with aging. This leads to heat intolerance because humans depend heavily on evaporative cooling. Decreased perspiration may be the result of decreased skin blood flow and loss of sweat glands. Physical activity should be limited or avoided in hot weather, particularly if it is humid. To maintain a program through the summer, you should exercise early in the morning before the heat sets in.

If you are older and undertake an exercise program, you will experience cardiovascular benefits just as younger people do. The response to endurance conditioning is slower in older people, but the benefits will come— those that can be measured and those that are intangible but important to daily living.

Be prepared for six or seven weeks to go by before you can measure an improvement in cardiac function. Other benefits will come more quickly. An increased feeling of strength and agility will be yours within two or three weeks. A daily commitment to some form of activity and a thrice-weekly commitment to cardiovascular conditioning will enable you to carry out work and recreation with less fatigue. That feeling of increased vigor will make these activities more enjoyable and make you a more enjoyable person to be with. Your social horizons will expand because you will become a more vital and outgoing person.

8

The Romance of the River

*I'm beginning to find what I sought when I started rowing—a sense of
self-worth, personal development, and CONFIDENCE—*
                                        Barbara Kirch, Diary, 1981.

The Growth of an Athlete
by Barbara Kirch

My most exciting moments in rowing come when I am so focused on
making the boat glide forward that I don't even feel how hard I am pulling. I am
being as powerful and explosive as I can be, but I am also focusing on being
effective, balancing on the fine edge between blind exertion and the right
amount of concentration to keep my body under control. The boat feels as if it is
barely skimming the surface of the water as it is being accelerated by the oars.
During moments like these I want time to stand still.

I am gifted with a strong, healthy body. Fortunately, with work, it has
allowed me to achieve the athletic goals of my dreams. Yet it did not start that
way. Because I was strong and well coordinated, I always learned sports quickly.
But a pattern developed in which I would excel quickly and then, in about a
year, plateau. I could not seem to rise above a certain level in any sport I
attempted. In frustration, I would imagine myself miraculously improving simply
because I wanted to so desperately. At the same time, though, I did nothing to
change my training regimen. The miracle never came. In fact, the more I hoped
my performances would improve, the more they declined.

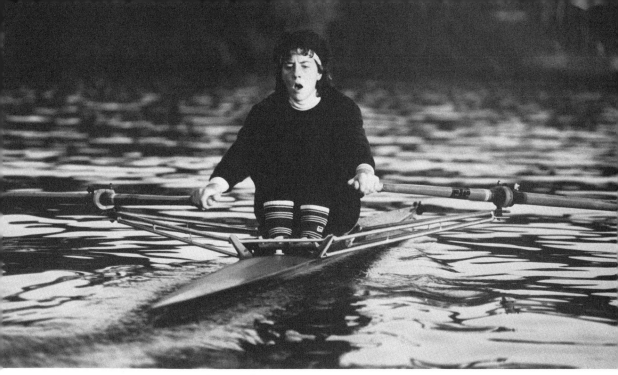

Barbara balanced at the catch.
The boat is twenty-seven feet long but no more than a sliver wide.

The answer? Keep switching sports? Try to find a sport where excellence is more easily achieved? Changing did not prove to be the solution. The plateau was always there and never surpassed. Because of my natural strength and coordination, I was not applauded for "heart" or for "extra effort." Instead, I was considered an athlete with potential—and just that. Potential without fulfillment means very little in sports. It means very little in anything, as I have discovered, unless you can prove that you are on the way to developing that potential. I began to see myself as lazy and as a failure—as someone unwilling to pay the price of pain to push my body past all the others who were working so hard.

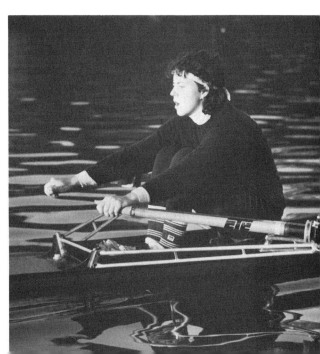

Deep down, I knew I had heart, and when the time was right, I would give everything I had to whatever I had chosen. But it didn't look as if I was ever going to find the sport that would motivate me or be important enough to me to push me over the hump of "potential" and on to growth—until I started rowing.

I "knew" from my first day on the water that I was going to grow with rowing. I felt completely at ease with other rowers. When I first walked into the boathouse, I felt at home. The people were very athletic—and attractive. Neither musclebound nor emaciated. Just all-American healthy looking. There was depth to their eye contact, and they spoke to each other with respect. They carried themselves with confidence.

"United States National Rowing Team." That patch was on about four different jackets. People started talking to me. I had the feeling that I had found my niche. I was light years away from their level of conditioning, but mentally I felt very comfortable with them. This was a diverse group of people, with more than just the sport to discuss. One was a bridge builder, another was in law school. Yet another was in business, still another was a carpenter. These seemed to be people who were successful at whatever they did.

I fit in physically, too. I felt about average in size, rather than being huge. I am 5'11". I used to hate my legs because they were bigger than other girls' and most boys'. Now I had found a sport that made them an asset. I soon loved what they could do.

I had never been to Boathouse Row before, yet I felt as if I had come home. I didn't know exactly where rowing was going to take me, but I decided on that first day to take learning one step at a time. I was in no hurry. I wanted to build a strong foundation that would hold up against the setbacks that would inevitably occur when I progressed. In this sport I was not going to plateau early, never to move forward. I had come into it stronger than most newcomers, yet there was much room for improvement. I loved the rowing motion, the water, being outdoors in all kinds of weather.

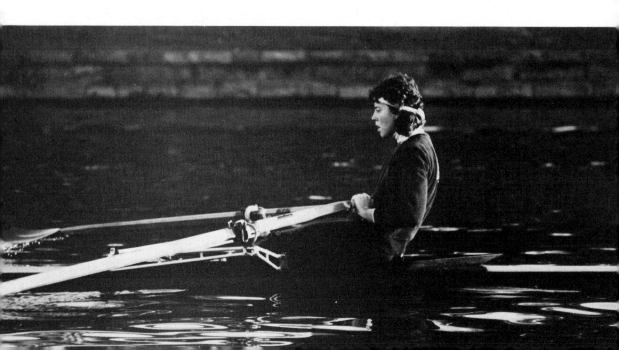

Within one month, I had progressed from a Gig (a wide, rowboat-like, learning boat) to a Quad (sculling—four people with two oars each), a double, and, finally, to a racing single.

I was told that I could row anything if I could master a single. Many miles of timid and terrified rowing passed under me in succeeding months. Having capsized three times in the first week of single sculling, I was somewhat leery of the stability of those 25-foot-long boats that were no wider than my seat. If I pulled unevenly on the oars or pulled one side more deeply through the water than the other, the boat would lurch to one side and I would assume that I was about to go for another swim. Fortunately, though, I would occasionally take one stroke just right so that the boat shot forward nicely balanced. The feeling was so exciting that I knew I couldn't quit. It had to be possible to take ten strokes in a row like that!

What fascinated me about rowing was that it required a combination of strength, endurance, and skill. It was a breakthrough for me because I could distract myself from pain and exhaustion by thinking about technique.

The rowing skills necessary to accommodate perpetually changing water conditions meant that each day would bring something new. Even though strokes were repeated hundreds of times, no two were ever exactly the same.

Without realizing it, my fitness level improved dramatically. It was fun to row a little bit farther each day while working on technique. I was amazed the first time that I rowed six miles. I had never covered that much distance under my own power before! I tried jogging again after about two months of rowing. I had never run a mile before without stopping. Two miles were gone before I thought about being tired. Was that miraculous? I certainly thought so.

Each day that I did a little more than I had ever done before, my confidence and excitement grew. Each day that I kept rowing when I was far from the boathouse, tired, lonely, and scared of flipping, I felt stronger. Something within me was changing.

After three months of rowing I was told that I had the "potential" to make the National Team in a year if I was willing to put forth a lot of effort. I was both thrilled and frustrated. The word "potential" struck a sore spot. To me, that statement meant that others thought I was still stuck on the same old plateau. I chose to ignore this inference because I was learning so much about myself through rowing. But I didn't forget it by any means. I had always dreamed of being a national or even an Olympic Team member, and I was not going to let someone's remarks be my reason for continuing. The actual sport of rowing was what kept me coming back.

For ten months of that first year, I sculled and trained in Hamburg, West Germany. It was there that I learned about soul-searching hard work as I trained with two members of the West German National Team. The only reason I didn't quit and just travel around Europe was that each time that I pushed myself to the point of tears in a workout, my performance improved. Sometimes I absolutely hated the work and the pain that went with it, but the improvements, small as they often were, were consistent. If I had quit then, I would have been satisfied

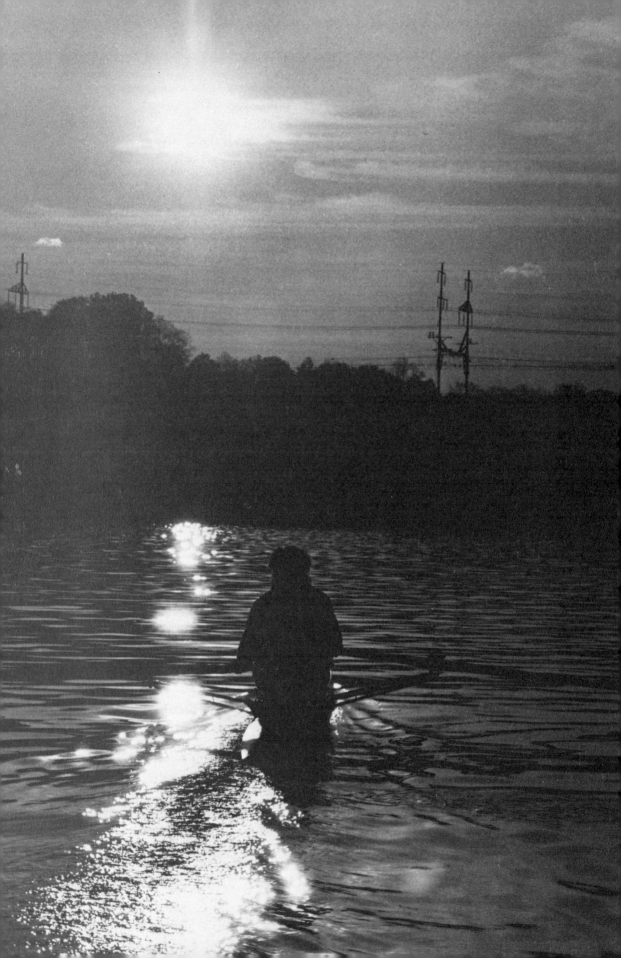

with my accomplishments, but how could I deprive myself of the opportunity to see just how far I could progress? I wanted to know just how good I could be.

An international race in Mannheim, West Germany changed my life. I was talking to my coach before the first heat. More than anything, I just wanted to go home and forget about competing. I was afraid of two things—pain and everyone else in the race.

I assumed that the other entrants had all trained just a little harder than I, or that they knew just enough more than I did to beat me. But had I ever trained this hard before? my coach asked. Was there anything more I could have done to prepare? I answered "no" to both questions, but was still scared. Why does someone else deserve to win any more than you do, he asked. I had no answer. We proceeded to discuss a race plan that dictated every single stroke I was going to take and how hard each would be. When I reached the 250 meters-to-go marker for the 1000 meter race, I was to close my eyes, grit my teeth, and pull as hard as I could.

At the starting line, adrenaline was flowing faster than blood in my veins. Why did I want to do this? I could be at home watching someone else do it on television. Germans, Danes, and Swedes surrounded me in the other five lanes. This was only the second time I had ever raced 1000 meters against more than one other person.

The starting command came in French as the flag went down. I was a little slow getting started, but I pulled as hard as I could for thirty strokes. Almost one-quarter of the race was over and I was still, amazingly, with the pack. Ten hard strokes left two people behind. Ten long strokes pulled me away from two others. At the halfway point I was dead even with one other person, and both of us were a boat length ahead of the rest.

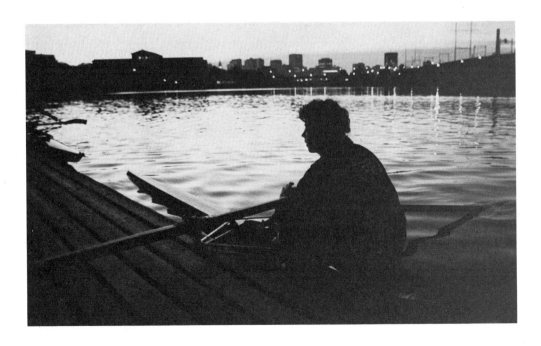

Another ten hard strokes, but we were still even. What did she know that I didn't? How had she trained that I hadn't? She pulled ahead by three-quarters of a length. The 250 meters-to-go mark was approaching. My legs were burning. What was so awful about coming in second? I was gulping for air. Two hundred and fifty meters to go—less than forty strokes.

Why does she deserve to win more than I? No answer. Then I went crazy. It was as if someone had flipped a switch in my head. I deserved to win because I had never worked so hard for anything in my entire life! I pulled blindly. My legs were driving so hard that they were numb. Thirty strokes to go. I moved up one-quarter of a boat length. Twenty strokes—she was only one-quarter length ahead. Ten strokes—it seemed even. The finish was determined by a photograph. She won by a bowball, a mere two inches.

But it didn't matter to me. I had won, too. Never in my life had I fought for myself like that. Never had I felt that I deserved something with enough conviction to pour everything I had into achieving it. I wasn't pushing myself to beat someone else. I pushed 110 percent because I deserved to win. The only feeling greater would be to give that much and win.

Since then, my finest achievements have always come when I started a race at a harder pace than I thought I could sustain, and then realized that I wanted and deserved a win badly enough to dig deep down inside and find a way to keep going at that pace or faster. I don't think a person can ever realize how much the body can do until she has had occasion to pull for her life.

Pull for my life I did to make the 1982 Penn Varsity Eight, the 1982 National Team Four with Coxswain, and then the 1984 U.S. Olympic Pair without Coxswain. Knowing what it takes to win does not always mean I am willing to do it. But now at least I realize the commitment involved.

Looking back, an Olympic athlete is really nothing more than a person with potential and a dream who has a few of the right doors opened. Someone said to me in 1980, "Here is the opportunity. You have the ability. If you are willing to put in the effort, it's yours. But you have a lot of work to do and no one can or will do it for you."

And as I learned to put forth 100 percent, people seemed to know and doors opened for me. I had changed from an athlete with potential to a real athlete. I was breaking all of my personal limits. I did not think of stopping. I wanted to keep going and find out how many more things I could discover about myself.

I had learned what many people later told me is true of achievement. If you want something to happen, you must make it happen yourself. Dreams are nice, but someone has to make them a reality. And that someone is you, or me, with simple hard work.

I still hate the pain that goes with training, when my muscles scream for oxygen and switching from one breath per stroke to two doesn't satisfy them. At the point where the body switches from aerobic to anaerobic metabolism, it's like going through a time warp, as the muscles scream for oxygen, the brain swears there is no more energy to be found, and then everything goes numb. This is probably the point many people call "the second wind." I dread reaching that point, but I am confident that my body will continue performing almost automatically.

As an athlete, fitness is my first concern. I give many hours each day to it, for without strength and endurance I could not excel in rowing. But there are other reasons for staying fit.

Cardiovascular fitness is the most important reason and applies to everyone, young or old, whether or not they are or have been athletic. Fitness can be achieved without athletic skill. It merely takes the commitment to spend a few hours a week in a motion vigorous enough to bring the heart rate to a level at which conditioning can take place.

Rowing is an excellent means to fitness. Whether on the water, in training facilities, or in people's homes, I see a variety of people using rowing for conditioning and recreation. I find this exciting. My own training includes work both on the water and off. In the winter, when the temperature drops into the teens and the chill factor is below zero, I find rowing on a straight pull ergometer in the warm shelter of the boathouse a pleasant and effective way to stay in shape. This type of machine very closely simulates the actual rowing motion.

Rowing is a growing sport. To familiarize you with it, we have included the following section describing the sport, its history, and some of the clubs and equipment that are available. A list of recreational and competitive boats is included. We hope that this will provide you with an appreciation of the sport of rowing, which has been prominent in the athletic history of the United States for more than a century.

The Evolution of the Sport

The Beginning—Rowing, now the epitome of amateur sport, began both in England and in America with professionals, men whose occupation it was to transport passengers and cargo across and along waterways in large, heavy rowboats. In 1715, to show appreciation for their efforts, British actor Thomas Doggett initiated an annual race for apprentice watermen on the Thames. The prize was an orange coat and a silver badge bearing the word "Liberty." This later became known as Doggett's Coat and Badge. Thus began the oldest continuous sporting contest in the world. Less than fifty years later watermen began racing in New York harbor at the urging of their own passengers. Rowing also flourished in other port cities such as Boston, Portland, and Philadelphia.

Through the middle and late nineteenth century rowing was the number one spectator sport in this country. Thirty thousand people lined the Charles River in Cambridge, Massachusetts, to watch a two-man race in 1877. Professionals, such as the Biglin brothers, the Wards, and James Hamill were considered the first real sporting heroes. They raced in singles, doubles, fours, and pairs for purses ranging from $50 to $3000, sizable sums for those times.

The Biglins and other oarsmen were subjects of Thomas Eakins' paintings. Thomas Eakins, who had many friends in the Philadelphia rowing

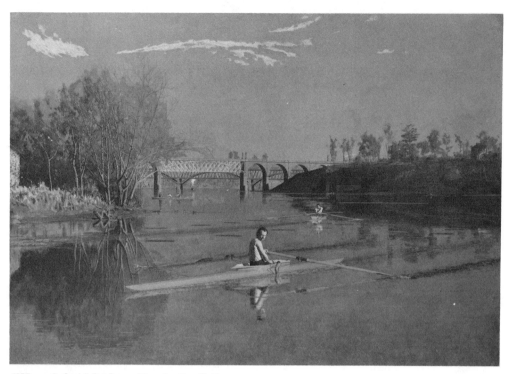

"Max Schmidt in a Single Scull."
(Painting by Thomas Eakins, 1871, The Metropolitan Museum of Art, Alfred N. Punnett Fund and gift of George D. Pratt, 1934.)

community, is said to have been an accomplished oarsman himself. The Thomas Eakins Head of the Schuylkill Regatta is held each October in Philadelphia. In England, too, artists gave their due to rowing. A distinct separation was made between amateur and professional athletes. There, the amateur rowers were depicted in very detailed, elaborate lithographs while professionals were captured in crude woodcuts.

Gambling played a part in the sport from its beginnings, and at times the outcome of a race was fixed through either equipment damage or bribery. An example of such chicanery was the series of three matches between arch rivals Canadian champion Edward Hanlan, winner of the Centennial Pro Race, and American rival Charles Courtney, winner of the Centennial Amateur Race, who had been undefeated in eighty-eight of eighty-eight amateur races. These races took place in the later 1870s following the Philadelphia Centennial Exposition of 1876, in which rowing and sailing were the only sports featured.

Each race was controversial—a trademark of professional rowing! Hanlan won the first race with a slower time than Courtney, because Courtney, though finishing first, disqualified himself by crossing lanes. Then, before the second race at Lake Chautauqua, New York, Courtney's boat was sawed in half. In the third race, Courtney stopped rowing two miles out with Hanlan well in the lead. The promoters of the event, manufacturers of a tonic called Hop Bitters, withdrew the $6,000 purse that had been promised to the winner.

By the turn of the century, professional rowing had declined, owing to the scandals surrounding so many events. But the popularity of rowing in the 1800s can be seen in statistics from the *Annual Illustrated Catalogue and Oarsman's Manual* of 1871 and the 1897 *National Association of Amateur Oarsman's Yearbook.* The former listed 237 clubs throughout the U.S., with 11,076 members. By 1897, with the decline of professional rowing, there were only 196 clubs. However, college crews were rapidly increasing in number. The United States Rowing Association was formed in 1873 and currently serves and represents amateur oarsmen and oarswomen in the United States, in 353 clubs.

Rowing began as a college sport in America in 1843 when a Yale junior purchased a secondhand Whitehall (similar to the American Star, the oldest existing racing boat) in New York for $29.50, with oars, and took it to New Haven to form the first American boat club at Yale. Rowing as a college sport had been established earlier in England, and the first Oxford-Cambridge Boat Race on the Thames had taken place in 1829. The race was 2¼ miles long and boasted a prize of 500 pounds. The Oxford boat can be seen in the South Kensington Science Museum in London.

Most of the boats racing up to this point were one, two, four, and six person craft. Harvard and Yale first promoted Eights. In 1876 Harvard and Yale posted the first intercollegiate race in America in Eights, over a course of four miles.

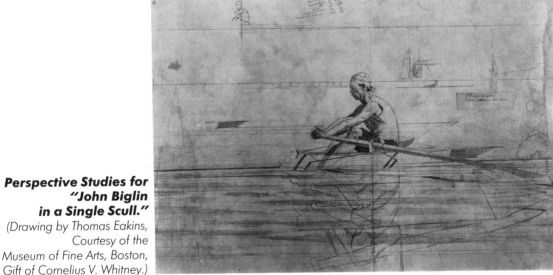

Perspective Studies for "John Biglin in a Single Scull."
(Drawing by Thomas Eakins, Courtesy of the Museum of Fine Arts, Boston, Gift of Cornelius V. Whitney.)

Harvard challenged Oxford for the first international amateur intercollegiate event, held on August 27, 1869 on the Thames. The American contingent included four oarsmen, a coxswain, two shells (Fours), a boat builder, two business managers, a cook, and a houseman. Upon arriving in England, they found the shells inadequate, and within a week the boat builder had constructed another boat. Publicity for this race equaled that of an Olympic event. There was front page coverage, complete with woodcut illustrations in *Ballou's Pictorial* and *Harper's Weekly* and details on the physical condition and stature of the athletes, their diets, and their training. Seven hundred fifty thousand people attended. Oxford won the match. The American rowers had suffered from travelers' illness and one oarsman got his oar tangled in his clothes during the race.

Although professional rowing died out, its impact can still be felt today. Many coaching tricks were kept secret during the professional era because of the high stakes of competition, but gradually, the knowledge and experience of the old pro's were utilized. Colleges and clubs frequently dissociated themselves from the professionals and tried to find what the British called "gentlemen-amateur coaches." Bob Cook, coaching at Yale from 1872 to 1896, filled this requirement, having means, leisure, and skill. His crews won fourteen of nineteen races. But former professionals gradually assumed a prominent role in amateur coaching. Charles Courtney, whose boat was vandalized at the Lake Chautauqua match, coached at Cornell from 1885 to 1919. His crews claimed 101 victories out of 146 competitions. Other universities, such as Syracuse and the University of Pennsylvania, also employed former professionals as coaches.

In the early days of English rowing there was a stronger dividing line between amateurism and professionalism than in America. Also, even into the 20th century, the sport was elitist and men who were laborers were barred from amateur competition because it was thought that their muscles gave them an unfair advantage over gentlemen. This was the reason ex-brickmason John B. Kelly was barred from entering the Diamond Sculls in 1920 at the Henley Royal Regatta on the Thames. Two months after the Henley, Kelly of the Vesper Boat Club took two Olympic gold medals, single and double sculls, and defeated the Englishman who had won the Diamond Sculls at Henley. Kelly won another gold

Sliders and sweep blades make patterns on the dock.

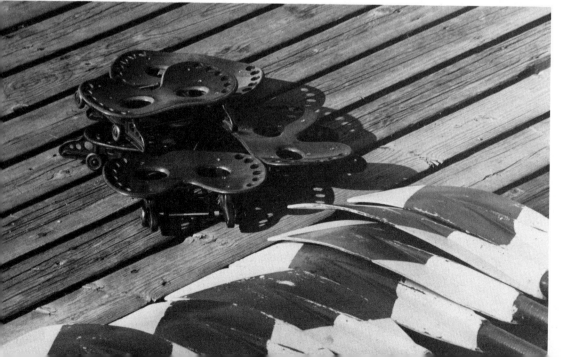

medal in the 1924 Olympics. In 1947 and 1949, his son John B. Kelly, Jr., won the Diamond Sculls at Henley. He also represented the U.S. Olympic team in single sculls in 1948, 1952, and 1956. John B. Kelly, Jr., died in March 1985, only a month after being elected president of the U.S. Olympic Committee.

Rowing style has evolved with changes in equipment. Before the advent of the sliding seat, the emphasis was on swinging from the hips with a straight back and rowing at a very high stroking rate. Then the six-inch slide under the seat allowed for the legs to get involved, although the upper body was still considered the source of power. The legs would initiate the stroke, followed by moving the upper body toward the bow, and ending with a quick pull of the arms. The recovery was led by the arms pushing down and away to clear the blade from the water. The boats in use were wide and heavy, and with the oars held on the gunwales by stationary wooden oarlocks.

This form of rowing was called English Orthodox, and was described in the first American book on rowing styles, *Principles of Rowing at Harvard.* Published by Harvard in 1873, it sold for 53 cents a copy. Technological advances in equipment necessitated certain changes from the English Orthodox style. A longer slide (twenty-seven inches) meant less body swing and more leg drive during the stroke. The legs had become the main power source. Swivel oarlocks on iron outriggers allowed the oar blade to be turned parallel to the water (feathered) to minimize wind resistance and allow the blade to skip off the water if it made contact. With the outriggers and the longer slide, the stroke was carried out on a horizontal plane rather than the more circular motion previously necessary to put the blades in the water for a solid stroke. This more horizontal motion became the American Orthodox style. In succeeding years, contact was maintained between the English and the Americans and changes were constantly being made to both styles.

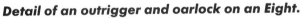

Detail of an outrigger and oarlock on an Eight.

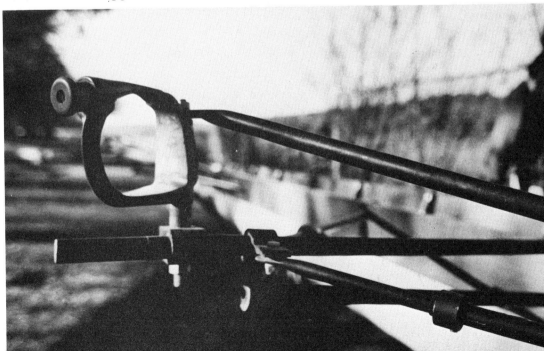

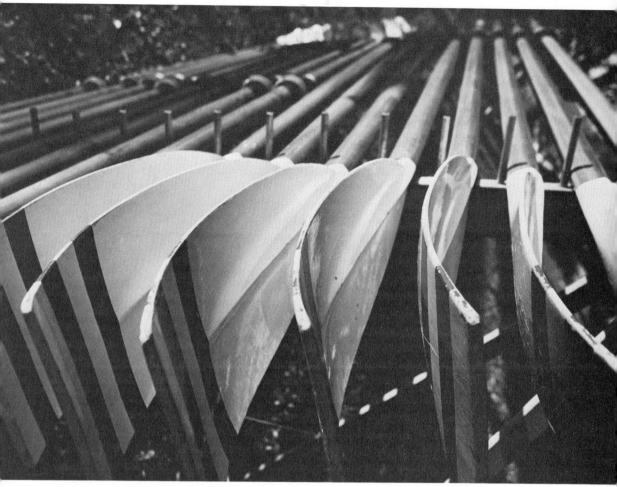

Racked sweeps, each twelve feet long, used with Pairs, Fours and eight-oared shells (i.e., one to a rower).

Training techniques evolved, too. Earlier, training consisted mainly of rowing six to seven miles each workout at about twenty-five strokes per minute. Some running was added to the program. This training was effective for the three- to five-mile races, which were the race lengths favored by the professionals in the early days. But with the advent of the shorter, 2000 meter (a mile and a quarter) event came the introduction of weight and interval training. Weight training increased strength. Interval training, designed to promote faster rowing for shorter periods, involved working harder in a workout for shorter periods, resting very briefly, then working again at high levels, barely allowing enough time to recover. This promoted increases in the body's ability to utilize oxygen.

Women's Rowing—Competitive rowing for women began in the late nineteenth century, which is now considered the golden age of rowing. Records indicate that the first women's rowing team was formed at Wellesley in 1877.

Among women, the competitive urge spread throughout the country. In 1888, Molly King, an oarswoman from Newport, Kentucky, challenged any female from Newport, Covington, and Cincinnati, to a two-mile race for stakes. The victory was to be decided on form rather than speed.

A few years later, a women's rowing club, ZLAC, was formed in San Diego, California. ZLAC stands for the first letters of each of the founders' names. Wearing high-necked full dresses, they rowed in men's barges, which were learning craft rather than shells.

The National Women's Rowing Association was formed in 1964. Championship races were 1000 meters long and international races were held. But it wasn't until 1975 that the first national selection camp and trials for the women's world championships were held. In 1976, women's rowing was introduced as an Olympic sport and Joan Lind won the silver for singles, and the U.S. eight won a bronze medal. Since that time U.S. women have done well in international competition, taking medals in all years since 1979. In the 1984 Olympics, the U.S. women's eight won the gold; the single, the silver; and the quad, the silver. All of the women's boats made the finals.

As of 1985, women race the same distance as the men, 2000 meters. 1985 will be the last year in which women will race 1000 meters in the U.S. Women's Nationals.

The Lure of the Sport—What draws people to rowing, either as a sport or as a means to stay fit long after competitive days are over? The training is arduous and painful. To stay with the sport weather must be ignored. Boston and Philadelphia, two of the largest centers of rowing, do not boast climates that are compatible with on-the-water activity year 'round. Why do people come to the river at 6 A.M. when it's cold and damp and go out for a row? And then go on to a full day's work or classes? Why does the novice never forget the first day on the water? The answers, of course, are individual. The lure of the sport can be very personal, but there are a few common reasons that keep coming up.

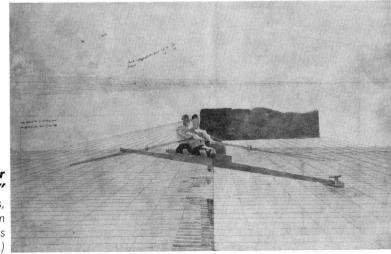

Perspective Drawing for "The Pair-Oared Shell."
(Drawing by Thomas Eakins, 1872, The Philadelphia Museum of Art, Purchased: Thomas Skelton Harrison Fund.)

Despite the hard work of rowing, it is compatible with the body. Unlike running, there is no pounding to the body. Water is soft. You can pull hard against it with the oar, but you will never feel the same jolt to your joints as when driving your legs against a sidewalk or a paved street. Rowing emphasizes smoothness and strength, and demonstrating these is satisfying. The entire body is involved in balancing and propelling the boat forward. From the catch to the recovery, the legs, arms, back, and stomach work together. When the oars have been put into the water, the body uncoils, shooting the boat forward. While the blades are out of the water, the body is coiling up again for the next stroke and again the boat glides smoothly forward. This rhythmic, graceful, energetic forward and back movement is entrancing. Also entrancing are the sounds. The blades splash a little as they slice into the water and then "whoosh" out of the water at the end of the stroke. When the boat is really moving fast, the water trickles along the hull like water moving over rocks in a stream.

Even the patterns made by the oars in the water are intriguing. It is a challenge to see how far the boat can move away from the little whirlpools left by the blades before the next stroke is taken, how many feet there are between whirlpools left by successive strokes. The object is to row the same number of strokes per minute while trying to get more distance between these "puddles" with each stroke.

The motion of a fast-moving boat is exhilarating. It seems to lift up out of the water, with perfect balance. This suspended feeling is so elating that rowers take special care to be smooth and to keep this sensation going as long as possible. At these moments pain and tiredness are dulled by the excitement of what seems to be perfection. If this feeling only lasts for ten strokes before the balance is lost, those ten strokes will not be forgotten. The thrill of the "perfect" stroke is so addictive that people row for years trying to recreate it.

While the rowing movement itself is appealing, a colorful sunset or a bright sunrise doubles the attraction of the sport. Every day the clouds and sky look different, and the air has a different feel. Though rowers do not always enjoy getting out of bed and trudging to the boathouse before dawn, there is a special sense of accomplishment or satisfaction when the sky begins to lighten halfway through a workout. Some enjoy knowing that they are getting a head start on their day and have the opportunity to see part of the day that most people miss.

Rowing means growth. It requires discipline. And it inspires dedication. But it also leaves room for many choices. It can be recreational or a lot of hard work. It can be a team or an individual sport. It provides an opportunity to push through mental and physical limitations, but does not insist upon it. Competitors row recreationally well after their bodies have peaked. It seems to be universally difficult to completely detach oneself from rowing after a few years—or even months—of regular participation. For all participants there is growth in rowing and a continuing sense of satisfaction.

Who are the Rowers?—People of all educational and occupational backgrounds are drawn to the sport. On the 1984 Women's Olympic Rowing Team, the "real life" occupations included physical therapist, musician, carpenter,

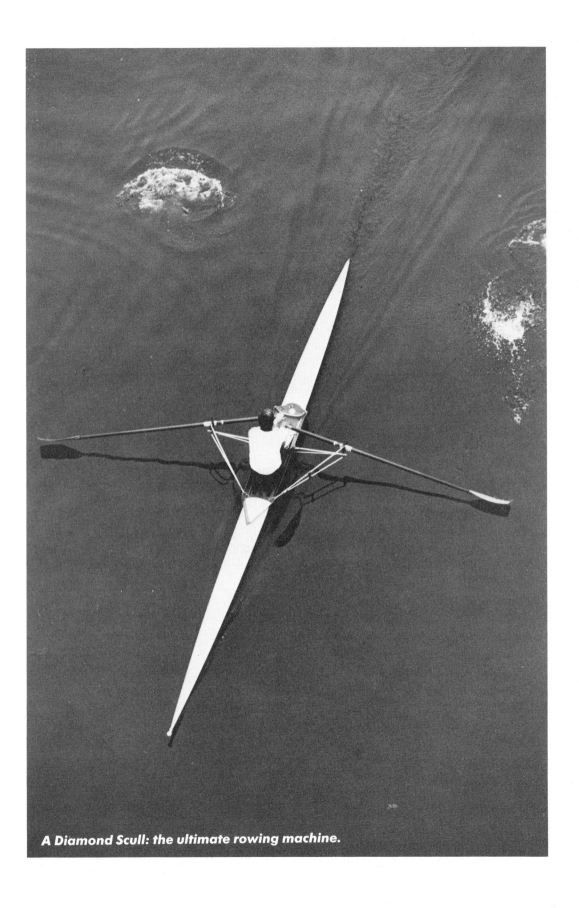

A Diamond Scull: the ultimate rowing machine.

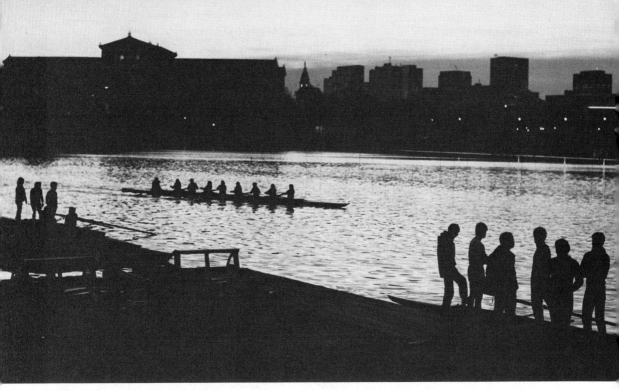

Coming in to boathouse row at dusk, with the Philadelphia Museum of Art anchoring the end of boathouse row on the Schuylkill.

physical education and special education teachers, pharmacologist, house cleaner, upholsterer, research assistant, student, hotel recreation manager, and bank teller. The men's team included some of these, as well as an investment banker, commercial fisherman, financial analyst, and a marine. College degrees had been earned in nutrition, biology, chemistry, English, business, physical therapy, music, law, and public health. This variety of occupations is seen in rowing at all levels. And then add to this the mix of age and physical attributes, and the variety of people multiply.

The United States Rowing Association (USRA) divides its membership into three competitive categories: Juniors, no older than eighteen by December; Regulars who are eighteen to twenty-six years old; and Masters, who are over twenty-six. In 1985 there were 1,781 Juniors, 6,634 Regulars, and 3,749 Masters registered with the USRA. Lightweight and heavyweight divisions are also recognized by the USRA in both men's and women's rowing. A lightweight woman weights 125 pounds or less, but in team boats, the average can be 130 pounds. Women 114 pounds and under are classified as flyweights. Lightweight men must weigh 160 pounds or less, with a boat average of 165 pounds. Any rowers over these weight limits are considered heavyweights.

In competitive rowing, the coxswain's seat is available to anyone weighing close to 120 pounds in the men's programs and 99 pounds in women's. A coxswain is the strategist, psychologist, and leader of the crew. His or her job is to steer the boat, make technical corrections, and guide the crew mentally and physically through workouts and races.

On the Schuylkill River in Philadelphia there are usually three groups of men and women of all ages participating in rowing programs: competitive, those rowing for recreation, and the handicapped (see following). Although rowing can be learned at almost any age, competitive rowing doesn't usually begin until about sixteen years of age. A well-developed muscular and cardiovascular system is necessary for high-level performance. Unless mature, the body doesn't reward high-intensity training with a high level of performance.

The competitive group rows for high school or college teams, or for the rowing clubs. In Boston, these line the Charles for three miles. In Philadelphia, they are in a small cluster on the Schuylkill called Boathouse Row. The tradition and history behind the sport can be felt by walking along the Row with its variety of buildings dating from the nineteenth century.

Recreational Rowing—A Growing Sport—Recreational rowing is growing as a means of fitness and relaxation. Now specially designed boats with sliding seats, but not so fragile, nor demanding as much skill, as the racing shells, are available for less than $1500. This is in contrast to a top-of-the-line racing single at $3,700. Recreational boats are wider than the racing shells, but still sleek enough for speed. Design emphasizes stability. The availability of these boats that has contributed to the growth of the sport. Those who would not dare to undertake rowing in a competitive shell, without good coaching and the willingness to take a dip or two now and then, can learn to use these recreational shells within a few minutes. They are light and easy to manage, both on and off the water. A list of suppliers and manufacturers of recreational rowing equipment can be found at the end of this book. A variety of these small craft can also be seen at boat shows.

Dick Dreissigacker (stroke) and Gordon Nash (bow) in competition with Small Craft Double, May 1984, Newport, Rhode Island.

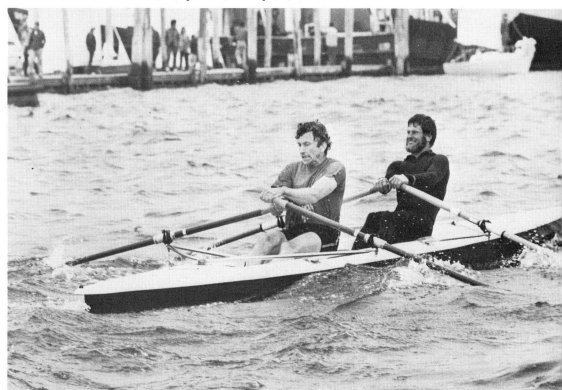

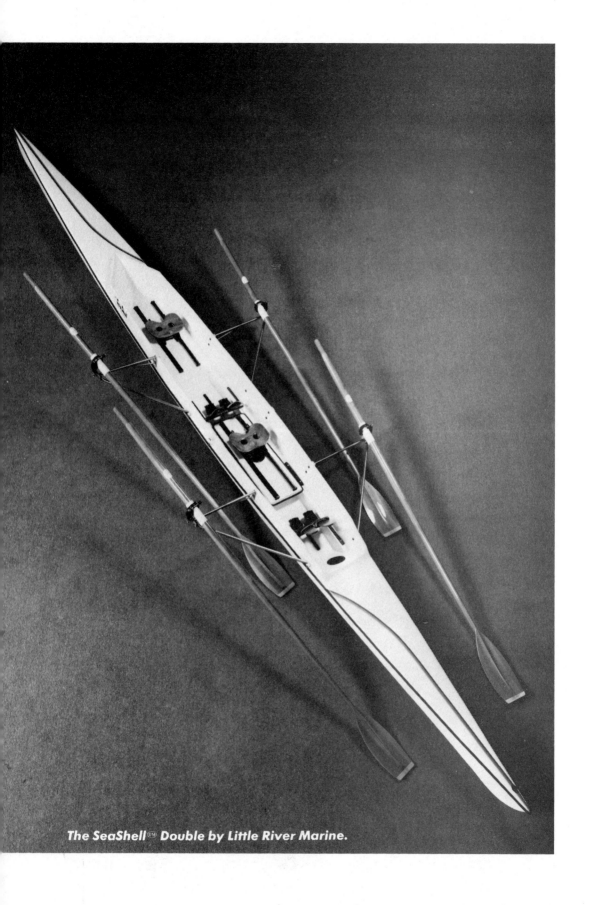

The SeaShell™ Double by Little River Marine.

Who are these recreational rowers? Very often they are fugitives from another sport, driven perhaps by the need to find a fitness medium that will not aggravate an existing injury. They universally report rowing as a thrilling means of fitness. The sensation of propelling the boat over the water is as addicting to these recreational rowers as to the competitive rowers. A major contributor to this sensation is the well-designed craft that is capable of responding in such an exciting way.

The other lure is that of the outdoors, and, of course, of the water. The lake, the inlet, the river, the bay, can be more than scenery with the right equipment. Of course, a shell, silently propelled, allows a perfect blending of man and nature.

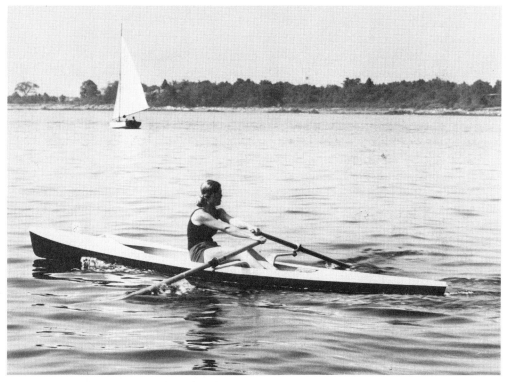

Liz Hills in Isles of Shoals Race in the Alden Ocean Shell Single with "Oarmaster."

Recreational, on-the-water rowing might be the step beyond the rowing machine for you. The cardiovascular fitness you have gained from your rower will translate well to the actual water sport, as will the strength in the large muscle groups. Your rowing machine will give you the physical conditioning needed to use a recreational shell on vacations, weekends, or when the weather is right. Once you get on the river you'll find yourself wanting to row on a more regular basis.

The Boats—There are two ways to row: sculling and sweep. "Sculling" is when each person in a boat has control over two oars, one on port, and one on starboard. One hand holds each oar, as in a lifeboat. The oars are about nine feet long. In "sweep" rowing, each person only has one oar, on either starboard or port, and both hands are used to control it. The oar is twelve feet long, and is heavier than the sculling oar. The smallest "sweep" boat is a Pair (two people) because at least one oar is needed on each side. The smallest sculling boat is a Single.

The Single is extremely sensitive. In a Single, it is just you, your boat, and the weather. Performance will depend on how well you use the combination. It is the perfect boat to row when trying to improve efficiency and technique because it reflects everything that the rower is doing. If rowed with strength and smoothness, it will glide forward with good speed. If the motion is rough and arrhythmic, the boat will move like a rocking horse through the water. It will stop and go as a bow dips down and then rises out of the water again. With good timing, the oars on both sides of the boat will enter and leave the water simultaneously and the boat will go straight forward and almost balance itself. Once this is mastered, the rower can relax and concentrate on rowing with energy, aggressiveness, and confidence.

The Double (sculling) or Pair (sweep) is also sensitive and can be used to refine technique for larger boats. The Double is an exciting, responsive, and quick-moving boat, and is easier to balance than the Pair. Because in the Double each rower controls two oars, all the force that they generate individually is applied to both sides of the boat. Even if the rowers are of differing strengths, the boat will still go straight. Not so with the Pair because each person is applying force to only one side of the boat. When one rower is stronger than another, the boat will gradually turn toward the weaker side. The Pair is like rowing a single with two people. Whatever the individual styles of the rowers, they must choose one and blend together.

The appeal of a two-person boat versus the single is companionship. There is an opportunity to work together to achieve the same result as with a well-moving single, but the work can be accomplished at greater boat speed. Also, a built-in support system exists. In fact, when two people train intensely together, they might occasionally feel almost "married." Perhaps they have come together with differing strengths and weaknesses to train for a particular race. Individually, they may be strong, but not fast enough to win. Together their abilities can add to a winning result. Because the success of the boat is dependent on the sum total of both efforts, Pair partners get to know each other so well that they often predict how the other is going to react to various rowing-related situations. Though their personal lives remain separate, they are seen as a single unit when on the water.

Four- and eight-person boats are not as spirited. Though they move faster through the water with their larger "engine rooms," they are longer, wider, and take more time to navigate turns. When the boat loses its balance, or "falls off keel," it happens more slowly than in a Single. With four or eight people balancing the boat, it is easier to make up for one person's falling off balance or lagging behind with a stroke.

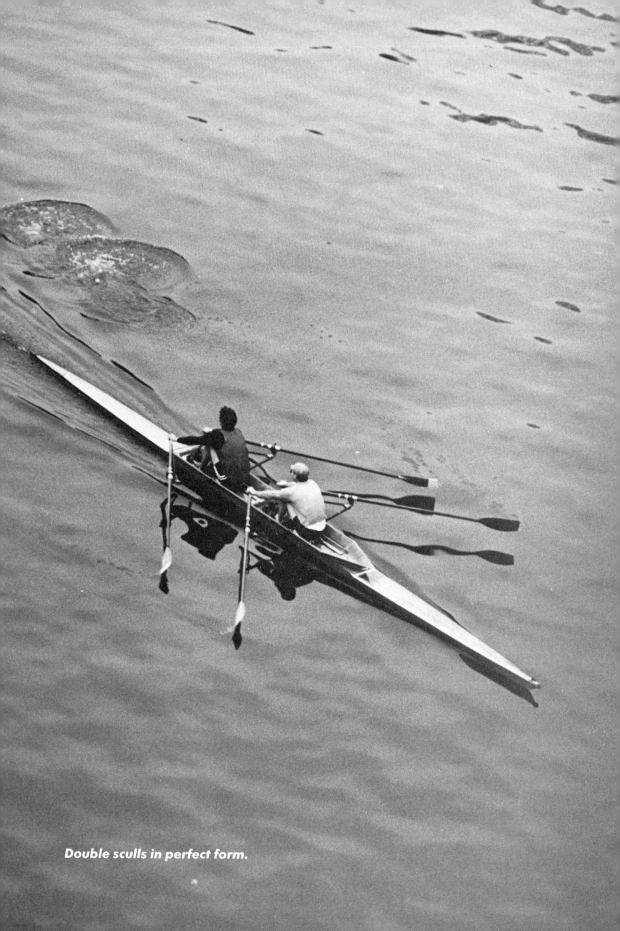

Double sculls in perfect form.

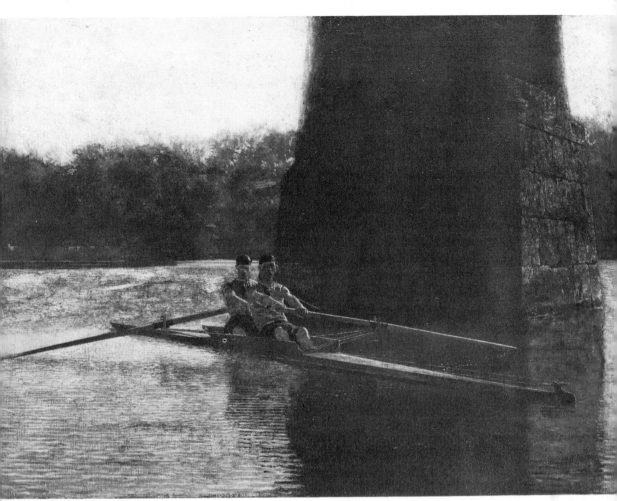

"The Pair-Oared Shell."
(Painting by Thomas Eakins, 1872, Philadelphia Museum of Art. Given by Mrs. Thomas Eakins and Miss Mary A. Williams.)

Looking up the course on the Schuylkill.

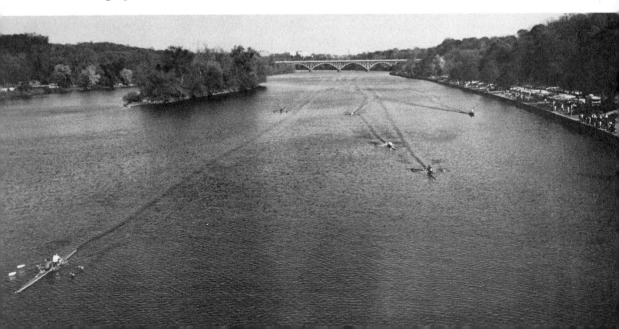

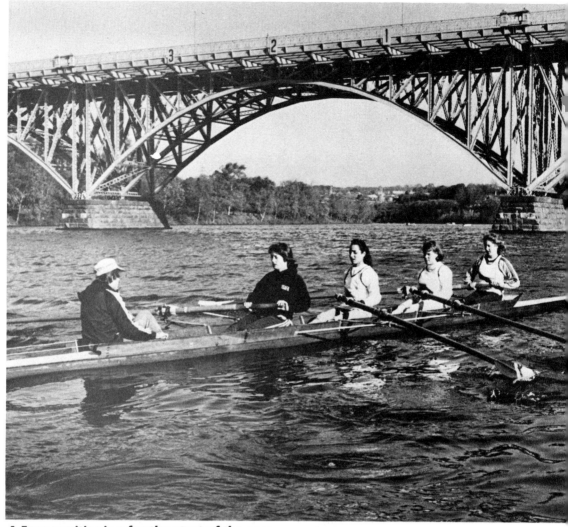

A Four positioning for the start of the race.

Rowing in a team boat is a nurturing experience. The energy from teammates makes it easier to get through hard workouts, and trying to blend with them distracts from the pain of the work. But then comes your customary quitting point! No one will stop and wait for you to catch your breath. And stopping yourself would blacklist you in the rowing world. The choice is stop and endure the wrath of the crew or keep going, pour your heart out, and maintain respect. Then there is the fact: if everyone else is able to keep rowing, it must be possible. So you go on. At the end of the workout, you will most likely find out you weren't the only one with thoughts of quitting. One grows through rowing by pushing through these limits.

Rowing a Four or an Eight is the ultimate team sport. There is no "Best Player" award. No one person in the boat gets any more credit than another for the boat's success. Yet each seat requires a slightly different talent. In an Eight, nine people can be world champions at the same time—eight rowers and the coxswain. Each is the star in his or her own position, but all work together for the win.

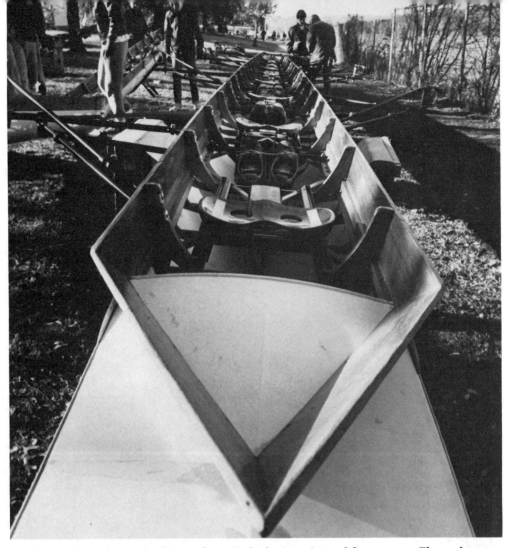

Looking down from the bow of an Eight being rigged for a race. These boats are about sixty-one feet long and eighteen inches wide.

A section of an Eight being rigged for a race. Fiberglass has replaced wood and hulls, have deepened somewhat over the last twenty years.

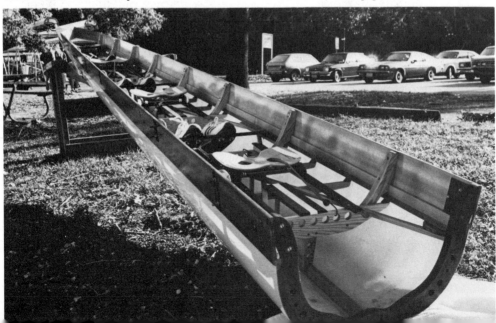

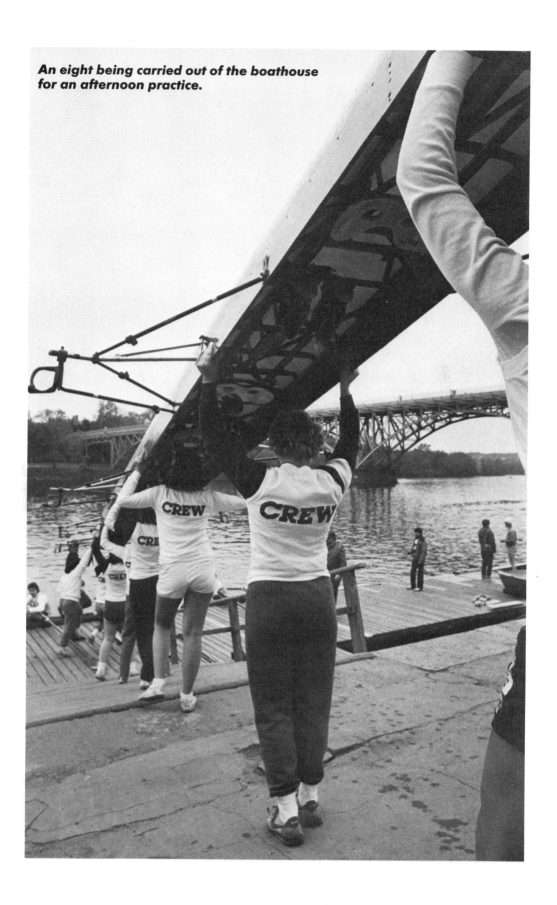

An eight being carried out of the boathouse for an afternoon practice.

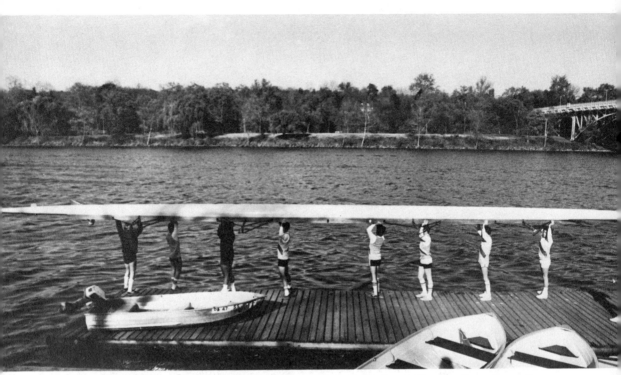

Getting a 61 foot boat in and out of the water is done "by the numbers," with the cox calling out each move.

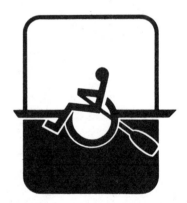

Freedom on the River—Rowing for the Disabled

About one mile upriver from Boathouse Row on the west shore of the Schuylkill River in Philadelphia stands the newly renovated boathouse of the Philadelphia Rowing Program for the Disabled (PRPD). Initiated in 1981 by Jim McGowan, a paraplegic, the PRPD provides recreational and competitive rowing for the physically and developmentally disabled. As of 1983, there were more than 100 rowers and a fleet of thirteen boats. The highlight of that season was the All Disabled Regatta on the Schuylkill, which attracted over 1000 able and disabled spectators. Participants in the PRPD have disabilities that include quadriplegia, paraplegia, amputations, cerebral palsy, spina bifida, hearing and visual impairments, and multiple sclerosis.

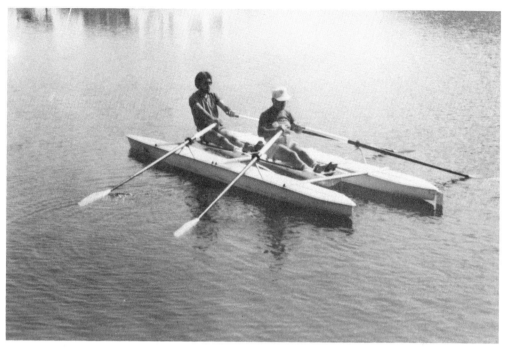

Randy Day of Omni-Cat and Chris Keim, seventy-eight.

The equipment used by members of the program has more stability than the boats used by the able-bodied competitive rowers. These include the Omni-cat, Row-Cat, and Alden shells. The boats come as Singles or Doubles and are supported by two pontoons, very much like catamaran sailboat hulls. Designed for balance and buoyancy, they are almost impossible to capsize. The Doubles are rowed by one disabled and one able-bodied rower for added safety and to provide opportunity for instruction. These boats can be adapted structurally according to the handicap of the user. The Alden boats have a single hull that is broader and more stable than the usual competitive shell and can be used by those who can use a sliding seat and who do not need the stability provided by the pontoons. In Philadelphia, the indoor training tanks at the University of Pennsylvania are used to help teach people to row before they venture out on the river. Indoor pools and rowing machines are also used. Row-Cat mitts, and other adaptive devices, make it possible for persons with impaired or absent muscle action in the wrists and arms to participate in rowing.

The value of rowing for the disabled is many-fold. Some of the benefits are the same as for able-bodied rowers, while others are special. Being outdoors, on the river, and propelling oneself forward with the same gliding motion as achieved by an able-bodied rower provides a sense of freedom not available to the disabled on land. There need be no wheelchairs or crutches, only a boat and two oars. With rowing, success is possible, and the feeling of accomplishment, satisfaction, and self-confidence achieved on the water can be transferred to other areas of life. As one rower, Bill Wright, puts it, "Each time you are out there, you do something you didn't do before."

The quiet beauty of the river, the sounds of the water and birds, and the

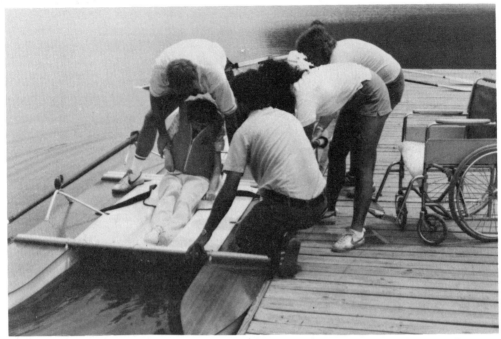

Disabled rower being assisted into an Omni-Cat at the Oak Ridge marina, Oak Ridge, Tennessee.

gentle gliding of the boat reduce tension and anxiety. Rowing increases endurance and stamina, improves the cardiovascular system, and enhances coordination and dexterity. Socially, camaraderie, repartee, and group spirit help overcome loneliness and provide a good time.

Leo Reilly is the current president of the PRPD. He is a below-the-knee amputee, blind, diabetic, and has had four kidney transplant operations. According to Reilly, "Boating helps the handicapped temporarily forget their disabilities and enjoy themselves. Also, the sport helps keep my diabetes under control. You build up your endurance out on the river. With my health problems, I'd have even more trouble if I didn't exercise."

Dolly Driscoll, now aged sixty, co-captain of the 1946 Radcliffe Women's Varsity Crew and later a biophysicist at Thomas Jefferson University, returned to rowing three years ago following a fall that left her a quadriplegic. Driscoll is a single and mixed double champion of the Freedom on the River Regatta, an all-disabled regatta held on the Schuylkill river.

As a quadriplegic who rows with her hands strapped to the oar handles, Driscoll says, "Rowing can be a rewarding exercise for most anyone, because you can use whatever muscles you have use of. It's just great being out on the river where you don't have to worry about curb cuts or manholes. In the spring, there are the cherry blossoms and the dogwoods. And you see the blue herons overhead."

The Freedom on the River program spread to Ann Arbor, Michigan, through the efforts of Doug Herland. Herland, who always dreamed of being a baseball player, was hindered by brittle bones. Herland was born with four broken ribs and a broken collarbone and pelvis, and only grew to the height of 4'8". A succession of broken bones before he was nine years old left him with one leg an inch and a half shorter than the other. He was manager and trainer for athletic teams all through high school. It wasn't until he started applying to colleges that it was suggested that he might be good as a coxswain in rowing.

Doug Herland learned to row a ingle in college. Though his legs were too weak to support his body, he found that by wrapping his knees he was able to row. As a result of this form of exercise, he was able to walk straighter and more comfortably because his atrophied hamstrings began to redevelop.

In bringing the Freedom on the River program to Michigan, Doug was able to share the "miracle" of rowing with others. Tom Komar, a quadriplegic, learned to row with him. When he realized that he was propelling the pontooned boat in a pool by himself, a look of wonder and disbelief spread over his face. Though his hands were tied to the oars and weights were put on his wrists to help him get the blades out of the water between strokes, no one was actually helping him. He describes the feeling as "unbelievable."

In June of 1984, Herland received a phone call asking if he would coxswain a Pair at the Men's Olympic Trials. He accepted and two months later he stood on the awards dock at Lake Casitas with an Olympic Bronze Medal around his neck. Rowing is a recent addition to the Special Olympics, but how many sports offer the opportunity for a disabled person to compete and win medals with the best able-bodied athletes in the world?

The most active rowing programs for the disabled at this time are in Ann Arbor, Michigan; Oakridge, Tennessee; and Philadelphia.

Programs for Disabled Rowers in the United States
(March 1984)

Philadelphia Rowing Program for the Disabled
Leo Reilly, Jr., Chairman
8800 Wissahickon Ave.
Philadelphia, PA 19128

Rowing for the Handicapped Program
c/o Chris P. Keim
102 Orchard Lane
Oak Ridge, TN 37830

Freedom on the River Program
c/o Mr. Douglas Herland
2567 Braiburn Circle
Ann Arbor, MI 48104

Mendota Rowing Club, Program for the Disabled
Attn: Kerstin Doell
2305 Park Street
Madison, WI 53713

Lake Meritt Rowing Club
Program for the Disabled
P.O. Box 1046
Oakland, CA 94604

Appendix A

Bibliography

The Exercise Initiative

1. Cooper, K.H.: Physical training programs for mass scale use: effects on cardiovascular disease—facts and theories. *Annals of Clinical Research* 14, Suppl. 34:25, 1982.

2. Leon, A.S., and Blackburn, H.: Physical inactivity. IN: *Prevention of Coronary Heart Disease: Practical Management of the Risk Factors.* N.M. Kaplan and J. Stamler (eds.) W.B. Saunders, Philadelphia, 1983.

Weight

1. Bray, G.A.: The energetics of obesity. *Medicine and Science in Sports and Exercise* 15:32, 1983.

2. Kukkonen, K., Rauramaa, R., Siitonen, O., and O. Hänninen: Physical training of obese middle-aged persons. *Annals of Clinical Research* 14. Suppl. 34:80, 1982.

3. Mandroukas, K., Krotkiewski, M., Hedberg, M., Wroblewski, Z., Björntorp, P., and Grimby, G.: Physical training in obese women. Effects of muscle morphology, biochemistry and function. *European Journal of Applied Physiology* 52:355, 1984.

4. McArdle, W.D., Katch, F.I., and Katch, V.L.: Obesity and weight control. (Chapter 28) *Exercise Physiology. Energy, Nutrition, and Human Performance.* Lea and Febiger, Philadelphia, 1981.

5. Morris, J.N., Everitt, M.G., Pollard, R., and Chave, S.P.W.: Vigorous exercise in leisure-time: protection against coronary heart disease. *Lancet* 2:1207, 1980.

6. Pauly, J.T., Palmer, J.A., Wright, C.C., and Pfeiffer, G.J.: The effect of a 14-week employee fitness program on selected physiological and psychological parameters. *Journal of Occupational Medicine* 24:457, 1982.

7. Paffenbarger, R.S.: Physical activity as a defense against coronary heart disease. (Chapter 8) IN: *Coronary Heart Disease: Prevention, Complications and Treatment.* W.E. Connor and J.D. Bristow (eds.) J.B. Lippincott, Philadelphia, 1985.

8. Paffenbarger, R.S., Jr., Hyde, R.T., Wing, A.L., and Steinmetz, C.H.: A natural history of athleticism and cardiovascular health. *Journal of the American Medical Association* 252:491, 1984.

9. Sullivan, L.: Obesity, diabetes mellitus and physical activity—metabolic responses to physical training in adipose and muscle tissues. *Annals of Clinical Research* 14, Suppl. 34:51, 1982.

10. Terjung, R.: Endocrine response to exercise. *Exercise and Sports Sciences Reviews* 7:153, 1979.

Cardiovascular Fitness

1. Blair, S.N., Goodyear, N.N., Gibbons, L.W., and Cooper, K.H.: Physical fitness and incidence of hypertension in healthy normotensive men and women. *Journal of the American Medical Association* 252: 487, 1974.

2. Cooper, K.H.: Physical training programs for mass scale use: effects on cardiovascular disease—facts and theories. *Annals of Clinical Research* 14, Suppl. 34: 25, 1982.

3. McArdle, W.D., Katch, F.I., and Katch, V.L.: Functional capacity of the cardiovascular system (Chapter 17). *Exercise Physiology: Energy, Nutrition, and Human Performance.* Lea and Febiger, Philadelphia, 1981.

4. Morris, J.N., Everitt, M.G., Pollard, R., and Chave, S.P.W.: Vigorous exercise in leisure-time: protection against coronary heart disease. *Lancet* 2:1207, 1980.

5. Paffenbarger, R.S.: Physical activity as a defense against coronary heart disease. (Chapter 8) IN: *Coronary Heart Disease: Prevention, Complications, and Treatment.* W.E. Connor and J. D. Bristow (eds.) J.B. Lippincott, Philadelphia, 1985.

6. Paffenbarger, R.S., Jr., Wing, A.L., and Hyde, R.T.: Physical activity as an index of heart attack risk in college alumni. Journal of Epidemiology 108: 161, 1978.

7. Paffenbarger, R.S., Jr., Wing, A.L., Hyde, R.T., and Jung, D.L.: Physical activity and incidence of hypertension in college alumni. Journal of Epidemiology 117:245, 1983.

8. Saltin, B., and Rowell, L.B.: Functional adaptations to physical activity and inactivity. *Federation Proceedings* 39:1506, 1980.

9. Scheuer, J., and Tipton, C.M.: Cardiovascular adaptations to physical training. *Annual Review of Physiology* 39: 221, 1977.

10. Thom, T.J., Kannel, W.B., and Feinleib, M.: Factors in the decline of coronary heart disease mortality. (Chapter 1) IN: *Coronary Heart Disease: Prevention, Complications, and Treatment.* W.E. Connor and J.D. Bristow (eds.) J.B. Lippincott, Philadelphia, 1985.

11. Tipton, C.M.: Exercise, training, and hypertension. *Exercise and Sports Sciences Review* 12:245, 1984.

Aging

1. Åstrand, P.O.: Human physical fitness with special reference to sex and age. *Physiological Reviews* 36:307, 1956.

2. Adams, G.M., and deVries, H.A.: Physiological effects of an exercise training regimen upon women aged 52 to 79. *Journal of Gerontology* 28:50, 1973.

3. Bassy, E.J.: Age, inactivity, and some physiological responses to exercise. *Gerontology* 24:66, 1978.

4. Chapman, E.A., deVries, H.A., and Swezey, R.: Joint stiffness: effects of exercise on young and old men. *Journal of Gerontology* 27:218, 1972.

5. Council on Scientific Affairs, Division of Personal and Public Health Policy, American Medical Association: Exercise programs for the elderly. *Journal of the American Medical Association* 252:544, 1984.

6. Ingebretsen, R.: The relationship between physical activity and mental factors in the elderly. *Scandinavian Journal of Social Medicine Suppl.* 29:153, 1982.

7. Laerum, M., and Laerum, O.D.: Can physical activity counteract aging? *Scandinavian Journal of Social Medicine Suppl.* 29:147, 1982.

8. Landin, R.J., Linnemeier, M.D., Rothbaum, M.D., Chappelaer, B.S., and Nobel, R.J.: Exercise testing and training of the elderly patient. In: *Exercise and the Heart*. N. Wenger (ed.) F.A. Davis, Philadelphia, 1984.

9. Saltin, B., Hartley, L.H., Kilbom, A., and Astrand, I.: Physical training in sedentary middle-aged and older men. II. Oxygen uptake, heart rate, and blood lactate concentration at submaximal and maximal exercise. *Scandinavian Journal of Clinical and Laboratory Investigation* 24:323, 1969.

10. Sidney, K.H., and Shephard, R.J.: Activity patterns of elderly men and women. *Journal of Gerontology* 32:25, 1977.

Program

1. Council on Scientific Affairs, Division of Personal and Public Health Policy, American Medical Association: Exercise programs for the elderly. *Journal of the American Medical Association* 252:544, 1984.

2. Drinkwater, B.L., and Horvath, S.M.: Heat tolerance and aging. *Medicine and Science in Sport* 11:49, 1979.

3. Gibson, S.B., Gerberich, S.G., and Leon, A.S.: Writing the exercise prescription: an individualized approach. *The Physician and Sportsmedicine* 11:87, 1983.

4. Kirkendall, D.T.: Exercise prescription for the healthy adult. *Primary Care* 11:23, 1984.

5. Leon, A.S., and Blackburn, H.: Physical inactivity. In: *Prevention of Coronary Heart Disease. Practical Management of Risk Factors*. N.M. Kaplan and J. Stamler (eds.) W.B. Saunders, Philadelphia, 1983.

6. Lombardo, J.A.: Preparticipation physical evaluation. *Primary Care* 11:3, 1984.

7. McArdle, W.D., Katch, F.I., and Katch, V.L.: *Exercise Physiology: Energy, Nutrition, and Human Performance*. Lea and Febiger, Philadelphia, 1981.

8. Pauly, J.T., Palmer, J.A., Wright, C.C., and Pfeiffer, G.J.: The effect of a 14-week employee fitness program on selected physiological and psychological parameters. *Journal of Occupational Medicine* 24:457, 1982.

9. Pollock, M.L.: The quantification of endurance training programs. *Exercise and Sports Sciences Reviews* 1:155, 173.

10. Shellock, F.G.: Physiological benefits of warm-up. *The Physician and Sportsmedicine* 11:134, 1983.

11. Smith, E.L.: Physical activity prescription for the older adult. *The Physician and Sportsmedicine* 11:91, 1983.

12. Wiktorsson-Möller, M., Oberg, B., Ekstrand, J., and Gillquist, J.: Effects of warming up, massage, and stretching on range of motion and muscle strength in the lower extremity. *The American Journal of Sports Medicine* 11:249, 1983.

Lipids

1. Hostmark, A.T.: Physical activity and plasma lipids. *Scandinavian Journal of Social Medicine Suppl.* 29:83, 1982.

2. Huttunen, J.K., Lansimies, E., Voutilainen, E., Ehnholm, C., Hietanen, E., Pentilla, I., Sittonen, O., and Rauramaa, R.: Effect of moderate physical exercise on serum lipoproteins: A controlled clinical trial with special reference to serum high-density lipoproteins. *Circulation* 60:1220, 1979.

3. Illingworth, D.R., and Connor, W.E.: Hyperlipidemia and coronary heart disease. (Chapter 2) In: *Coronary Heart Disease. Prevention, Complications and Treatment.* W.E. Connor, and J.D. Bristow (eds.) J.B. Lippincott, Philadelphia, 1985.

4. Miller, G.J., and Miller, N.E.: Plasma high-density lipoprotein concentration and development of ischaemic heart-disease. *Lancet* 1:16, 1975.

5. Nakamura, N., Uzawa, H., Maeda, H., and Inomoto, T.: Physical fitness. Its contribution to serum high density lipoprotein. *Atherosclerosis* 48:173, 1983.

6. Wood, P.D., and Haskell, W.L.: The effect of exercise on plasma high density lipoproteins. *Lipids* 14:417, 1979.

7. Wood, P.D., Haskell, W.L., Blair, S.N. Williams, P.T., Lindgren, F.T., Albers, J.J., Ho, P.H., and Farquhar, J.W.: Increased exercise level and plasma lipoprotein concentrations: a one-year, randomized, controlled study in sedentary, middle-aged men. *Metabolism* 32:31, 1983.

Metabolism

1. LeBlanc, J., Tremblay, A., Richard, D., and Nadeau, A.: Daily variations of plasma glucose and insulin in physically trained and sedentary subjects. *Metabolism* 32:552, 1983.

2. Terjung, R.: Endocrine response to exercise. *Exercise and Sports Sciences Reviews* 7:153, 1979.

3. Tremblay, A., Nadeau, A., and LeBlanc, J.: The influence of high carbohydrate diet on plasma glucose and insulin of trained subjects. *European Journal of Applied Physiology* 50:155, 1983.

Romance

1. Anne Cassidy: The comeback of Dolly D. *McCall's,* November, 1983.

2. Greenstine, J.: Freedom on the River Regatta. *Sports 'n Spokes* July/August, 1983.

3. McMillan, C.: Rowing regatta. *USAIR,* October, 1984.

4. Mendenhall, T.C.: *A Short History of American Rowing.* Charles River Books, Boston.

5. Robbins, W.: In Philadelphia, scullers arise before crocuses. *The New York Times,* March 26, 1982.

6. Stoler, P.: The solitary joys of sculling. *The New York Times Magazine,* July 24, 1983.

7. Wellemeyer, M.: On your own time. *Fortune,* April 20, 1981.

8. Rowing/Olympics. An exhibition organized by J. David Farmer. University Art Museum, University of California, Santa Barbara. 20 June—5 August 1984 (catalog)

Psychology

1. Benson, H.: *The Mind/Body Effect.* Simon and Schuster. New York, 1979.

2. Eide, R.: The effect of physical activity on emotional reactions, stress reactions, and related physiological reactions. *Scandinavian Journal of Social Medicine Supplement* 29:103, 1982.

3. Eide, R.: The relationship between body images, self-image and physical activity. *Scandinavian Journal of Social Medicine Supplement* 29:109, 1982.

4. Massie, J.F., and Shephard, J.R.: Physiological and psychological effects of training—a comparison of individual and gymnasium programs, with a characterization of the exercise drop-out. *Medicine and Science in Sports and Exercise* 3:110, 1971.

5. Morgan, P.W.: Anxiety reduction following acute physical activity. *Psychiatric Annals* 9(3):36, 1979.

6. Rossi, B., and Zoccolotti. Body perception in athletes and nonathletes: *Perceptual and Motor Skills* 49:723, 1979.

7. Sonstroem, R.J.: Exercise and self-esteem. *Exercise and Sports Sciences Reviews* 12:123, 1984.

8. Wilson, V.E., Vietta, B.G., and Bird, I.E.: Effects of running and of an exercise class on anxiety. *Perceptual and Motor Skills* 53:472, 1981.

9. Wilson, V.E., Morley, N.C., and Bird, E.I.: Mood profiles of marathon runners, joggers and nonexercisers. *Perceptual and Motor Skills* 50:117, 180.

Nutrition and Physiology

1. Berne R.M., and Levy, M.N.: *Cardiovascular Physiology,* 4th ed. C.V. Mosby, St. Louis, 1980.

2. V.P. Mountcastle, ed.: *Medical Physiology,* 14th ed. C.V. Mosby, St. Louis, 1980.

3. Smith, N.A.: Nutrition and athletic performance. *Primary Care* 11(1):33, 1984.

4. Smith, N.A.: Nutrition and the athlete. *Orthopedic Clinics of North America* 14(2):387, 1983.

5. Consolazio, C.F.: Nutrition and performance. *Progress in Food and Nutrition Science* 7:187, 1983.

6. J.C. Breneman, ed.: *Basics of Food Allergy,* 2nd ed. Chas. C. Thomas, Springfield, Ill., 1984.

7. Appenzeller, O., and Atkinson, R., eds.: *Sports Medicine: Fitness, Training, Injuries.* Urban and Schwartzenberg, Baltimore, 1981.

8. Bassler, T.J.: Hazards of restrictive diets. *Journal of the American Medical Association* 252(4):483, 1984.

Appendix B

Sports Medicine Centers

This list is not intended to be a comprehensive directory of sports medicine centers in the United States, nor should inclusion in this list be construed as an endorsement. We suggest that in making a contact, you explain your needs and then determine if a given facility is appropriate for you. You may also contact any of the centers listed below for referrals to physicians or other centers in your locality.

University Hospital Heart Station
University of Alabama
Birmingham, Alabama 35294

The Sports Medicine Clinic
Phoenix Sports Medicine
and Orthopedics
1950 W. Heatherrae
Phoenix, Arizona 85015

Tucson Sports Medicine Clinic
St. Mary's Medical Park
1779 W. St. Mary's Road
Tucson, Arizona 85745

CVR Fitness Clinic
Box 2507
University of Arkansas
Monticello, Arkansas 71655

National Athletic Health Institute
575 E. Hardy Street
Inglewood, California 90301

Douglas W. Jackson, M.D.
2760 Atlantic Avenue
Long Beach, California 90806

Center for Sports Medicine
St. Francis Memorial Hospital
900 Hyde Street
San Francisco, California 94109

Steven I. Subotnick DPM, MS
19682 Hesperian Blvd.
Hayward, California 94541

Crowl Sports Injury Center
5207 J Street
Sacramento, California 95819

Fort Collins Sports Medicine Clinic
1148 E. Elizabeth Street
Fort Collins, Colorado 80524

New Haven Sports Medicine Center
St. Raphael Hospital
Chapel Street
New Haven, Connecticut 06511

Cardiac Rehabilitation Program
George Washington University
Smith Center
22nd and G Street, N.W.
Washington, DC 20052

Sports Medicine Clinic, PC
615 Peachtree Street, N.E.
Atlanta, Georgia 30308

Sports Medicine Education Institute, Inc.,
and Northside Sports Medicine Center
993 Johnson Ferry Road, N.E.
Atlanta, Georgia 30342

Northwestern University Medical School
Sports Medicine Clinic
303 E. Chicago Avenue
Chicago, Illinois 60611

Cardiac Rehabilitation and
Health Enhancement Center
Swedish Covenant Hospital
5145 N. California Avenue
Chicago, Illinois 60625

Center for Sports Medicine and
Health Fitness
4911 Executive Drive
Peoria, Illinois 61614

Saint Joseph's Medical Center
Sportsmedicine/Health Awareness
811 E. Madison Street
South Bend, Indiana 46634

University of Iowa
Sports Medicine Services
Carver Pavillion
University of Iowa Hospitals and Clinics
Iowa City, Iowa 52242

Research Laboratory
Dept. of HPER
Seaton Blvd.
University of Kentucky
Lexington, Kentucky 40506

Sports Medicine and Physical Fitness
Center
University of Maryland
College Park, Maryland 20742

Berkshire Sports Medicine Institute
Adams Road
Williamstown, Massachusetts 01201

Sports Medicine Clinic
University of Mass. Medical Center
55 Lake Avenue N.
Worcester, Massachusetts 01605

Sports Medicine Clinic
Massachusetts General Hospital
Fruit Street
Boston, Massachusetts 02144

Sports Medicine Division
Children's Hospital Medical Center
300 Longwood Avenue
Boston, Massachusetts 02115

Boston University Sports Medicine
75 E. Newton Street
Boston, Massachusetts 02118

William Beaumont Hospital
Cardiac Rehabilitation Center
3601 W. 13-Mile Road
Royal Oak, Michigan 48072

Michigan State University
Sports Medicine Clinic
Clinic Center
138 Service Road
East Lansing, Michigan 48824

St. Louis Orthopedic Sports Medicine
Clinic
14377 Woodlake Drive, Suite 311
Chesterfield, Missouri 63017

Southwest Missouri Regional
Sports Medicine Clinic
Southwest Missouri State University
Springfield Missouri 65804

Human Performance Laboratory
University of Montana
Missoula, Montana 59812

Sports Medicine Center
University Hospital
100 Bergen Street
Newark, New Jersey 07103

Institute of Medicine in Sports
Hamilton Hospital
Box 2621
Hamilton Township, New Jersey 08609

Sports Medicine Clinic
Hospital for Special Surgery
535 E. 70th Street
New York, New York 10021

University Sports Medicine Service
Dept. of Orthopedic Surgery
Upstate Medical Center
550 Harrison Center
Harrison Street
Syracuse, New York 13202

Athletic Injury Treatment Center
University of Rochester Medical Center
601 Elmwood Avenue
Rochester, New York 14642

Cleveland Clinic
9500 Euclid Avenue
Cleveland, Ohio 44106

Cincinnati Sportsmedicine and
Orthopedic Center
1 Lytle Place
Cincinnati, Ohio 45202

Division of Sports Medicine
Oklahoma University Health Sciences
Center
Oklahoma City, Oklahoma 73190

Hamot Sports Medicine Center
Dept. of Physical Rehabilitation
Hamot Medical Center
Erie, Pennsylvania 16550

Harrisburg Area Sports
Medicine Center
3916 Trindle Road
Camp Hill, Pennsylvania 17011

Pennsylvania State Sports
Medicine Center
Milton S. Hershey Medical Center
Hershey, Pennsylvania 17033

Williamsport Hospital
Sports Medicine Center
777 Rural Avenue
Williamsport, Pennsylvania 17701

Temple University
Sports Medicine Center
Executive Plaza
540 Pennsylvania Avenue
Fort Washington, Pennsylvania 19034

Human Performance Laboratory
Holy Redeemer Hospital
1648 Huntingdon Park
Meadowbrook, Pennsylvania 19046

University of Pennsylvania
Sports Medicine Center
Weightman Hall E-7
235 S. 33rd Street
Philadelphia, Pennsylvania 19104

Human Performance Laboratory
Dept. of Physical Education, Health and
Recreation
University of Rhode Island
Kingston, Rhode Island 02881

Human Performance Laboratory
Physical Education Center
University of South Carolina
Columbia, South Carolina 29208

Cooper Clinic
12200 Preston Road
Dallas, Texas 75230

Sid W. Richardson Institute for
Preventive Medicine
Methodist Hospital
Texas Medical Center
6565 Fanin Street, Mail Station S-400
Houston, Texas 77030

Vienna Physical Therapy Association
501 Church Street
N.E. Suite 110
Vienna, Virginia 22180

Virginia Sportsmedicine Institute
1715 N. George Mason Drive
Arlington, Virginia 22203

Center for Sports Medicine
National Hospital for Orthopedics and
Rehabilitation
2455 Army Navy Drive
Arlington, Virginia 22206

Division of Sports Medicine
University of Washington
242 Hec Edmundson Pavilion
Seattle, Washington 98195

University of Wisconsin
Clinical Science Center
600 Highland Avenue
Madison, Wisconsin 53792

Orthopedic and Sports Physical Therapy
2501 Shelby Road
La Crosse, Wisconsin 54601

Appendix C
Recreational Rowing Crafts—Manufacturers and Suppliers

Caspian Boat Co.
P.O. Box 554
Manistee, MI 49660
(616) 723-9766
(616) 723-5106

Chicago Water Sports, Inc.
400 E. Randolph Street
Suite 2527
Chicago, IL 60601
(312) 938-1093

Composite Engineering, Inc.
Van Dusen Racing Boats
742 Main Street
Winchester, MA 01890
(617) 721-2156

Tom Donohoe and Co.
1606 Church Street
Decatur, GA 30033
(404) 292-1400

Durham Boat Company
RFD #2 Newmarket Road
Durham, NH 03824
(603) 659-2548

R. E. Graham Corp.
2601 E. Chapman Avenue
P.O. Box 2278
Orange, CA 92669
(714) 532-2085
and
Rt. 2, #2351 Hwy. 28
Quincy, WA 98848
(800) 572-6012

Hurka National Laboratories
41WO42 Colson Drive
St. Charles, IL 60174

Bill Knecht
P.O. Box 1346
Camden, NJ 08105
(609) 966-3636

Laser West
1769 Placentia Avenue
Costa Mesa, CA 92627
(714) 650-3080

Little River Marine Co.
PO Box 12722
Gainesville, FL 32604
(904) 378-5025

Lowell's Boat Shop, Inc.
459 Main Street
Amesbury, MA 01913
(617) 388-0162

Malia Kai Rowing Crafts
P.O. Box 5639
Kailua-Kona, HI 96740
(808) 329-3960

Martin Marine Co.
Box 2510, Goodwin Road
Kittery Pt., ME 03905
(207) 439-1507

Maumee Bay Boating Co.
5771 Bay Shore Road
Oregon, OH 43616
(419) 693-0636

Murphy Racing Shells
1728 N. 2nd Street
Minneapolis, MN 55411
(612) 588-9047

Omni-Cat Designs
715 Emory Valley Road
Oak Ridge, TN 37830
(615) 483-4387

Onion River Boat Works
Waterbury Ctr., VT 05677
(802) 244-6495

Orova Racing Shells
#4 Boathouse Row
Philadelphia, PA 19130
(215) 763-4250

Owen Racing Shells
P.O. Box 1167
Sisters, OR 97759
(503) 549-7702

Peinert Boatworks
52 Coffin Avenue
New Bedford, MA 02746
(617) 990-0165

George Pocock Racing Shells
509 NE Northlake Way
Seattle, WA 98105
(206) 633-1038

River Specialties, Lt.
19 Goldsborough Street
Easton, MD 21601
(301) 822-6233

The Row House
4 Maple Grove
Westport, CT 06880
(203) 222-0055/277-0008

Rowing Crafters
520 Waldo Point
Sausalito, CA 94965
(415) 322-3577

Sailing Systems
937 Mandarin Isle
Ft. Lauderdale, FL 33315
(305) 523-9343

Small Boat Gallery
48 Garrett Road
Upper Darby, PA 19082
(215) 352-9595

Small Craft, Inc.
P.O. Box 766
Baltic, CT 06330
(203) 822-8269

Surf and Offshore Sailing
1008 Richmond Avenue
Pt. Pleasant Beach, N.J. 08742

Tesco Products Corp.
1141 Penn Avenue
Wyomissing, PA 19610
(215) 375-7392

John Wright Boats, Inc.
1000 New De Haven Street
West Conshohocken, PA 19428
(215) 825-6610

Appendix D

Rowing Clubs and Organizations

Northeast

Alden Ocean Shell Assoc.
Ernestine Bayer
371 Washington Road
Rye, NH 03870

Alte Achter Boat Club
Peter Raymond
54 Creighton Street
Cambridge, MA 02140

Amherst College R.A.
Att: Crew Coach
Alumni Gym
Amherst College
Amherst, MA 01002

Amoskeag Rowing Club
95 Market Street
Manchester, NH 03101

Aqueduct Rowing Club, Inc.
2855 Aqueduct Road
Schenectady, NY 12309

Arlington High School
Crew
Att: Crew Coach
North Campus, Route 55
Pleasant Valley, NY 12569

Beach Channel High
School Crew
c/o William Stein
100-00 Beach Channel
Drive
Rockaway Park, NY 11694

Belmont Rowing Assoc.
Tim Wood
350 Prospect Street
Belmont, MA 02178

Berkshire School R.A.
Jack Stewart, AD
Route 41
Sheffield, MA 02157

Blood Street Sculls
Fred Emerson
RFD #3, Blood Street
Old Lyme, CT 06371

Boston University
Att: Crew Coach
285 Babcock Street
Boston, MA 02215

Brooks School Crew
Att: David T. Swift
1160 Great Pond Road
N. Andover, MA 01845

Brown Rowing Association
Norm Alpert
838 Greenwich Street #5F
New York, NY 10014

Brown University
Steve Gladstone
Box 1932, Athletic Dept.
Providence, RI 02903

Buckingham Browne &
Nichols
attn. C.W. Putnam
Gerry's Landing Road
Cambridge, MA 02138

Cambridge Boat Club
Gerry's Landing Road
Cambridge, MA 02138

Cascadilla Boat Club Ltd.
Eric Dicke, VP of CBC
106 Westfield Drive
Ithaca, NY 14850

Charles River R.A.
Harry Parker
60 J.F. Kennedy
Cambridge, MA 02138

Charter Oak Rowing Club
Harmon Leete
16 Sycamore Road
West Hartford, CT 06117

Choate Rosemary Hall
Crew
B.F. Sylvester, Jr.
Choate/Rosemary Hall
Box 788
Wallingford, CT 06492

Clark University
Att: Crew Coach
950 Main Street
Worcester, MA 01610

Colby College Rowing
Assoc.
Nancy Steck
Box 1609
Waterville, ME 04901

Colgate Rowing Club
Huntington Gym,
Colgate Univ.
Univ. Club Sports
Hamilton, NY 13346

College of the Holy Cross
Att: Crew Coach
Holy Cross College
Worcester, MA 01610

Columbia University
Ted Bonanno, Crew
Dodge Phy. Fitness Ctr.
New York, NY 10027

Conn. Rowing & Boating
Society
Todd Hudson, Pres.
12 A Dayton Court
Newington CT 06111

Connecticut College R.A.
Connecticut College
Box 1582
New London, CT 06320

Cornell University Crew
Att: Findlay Meislahn
Teagle Hall—P.O. Box 729
Ithaca, NY 14850

Craftsbury Sculling Center
Att: Crew
P.O. Box 31
Craftsbury Common, VT
05827

Dartmouth Rowing Club
301 Alumni Gym
Dartmouth College
Hanover, NH 03755

Durham Boat Club
Jim Dreher
RFD #2 Newmarket Rd.
Durham, NH 03824

E.A.R.C.
Att: Crew
P.O. Box 3
Centerville, MA 02632

East River Rowing Club
Will Waggaman
300 East 74th Street
New York, NY 10021

Exeter Boat Club
Att: Crew
Phillips Exeter Academy
Exeter, NH 03833

Exeter Rowing Association
Richard Tobin
11 Hall Place
Exeter, NH 03833

Fordham Rowing
Association
Att: Crew
Lombardi Mem. Ctr.
Fordham University
Bronx, NY 10458

Groton School
David Rogerson, Ath. Dir.
Farmer's Row
Groton, MA 01450

Hamilton Crew
Christopher J. Daniels
Hamilton College Box 1241
Clinton, NY 13323

Hanover Rowing Club
301 Alumni Gym
Dartmouth College
Hanover, NH 03755

Hartford Barge Club
Wayne Hobin
36 Country Lane
East Hampton CT 06424

Harvard Business School
B.C.
Student Assoc. Office
Kresge/Harv. Business
School
Boston, MA 02163

Harvard Law School Crew
Dean of Students
Harvard Law School
Cambridge, MA 02138

Harvard University
Att: Harry Parker
60 J.F. Kennedy
Cambridge, MA 02138

Head of the Conn. Regatta
P.O. Box 1
70 College Street
Middleton, CT 06457

Hobart & Wm. Smith R.C.
Carroll Driscoll
Box 188
Geneva, NY 14456

Housatonic Rowing Assoc.
Anne C. Boucher
81 Dana Street
West Haven, CT 06516

Hyde Park Rowing Assoc.
David Vertullo, Coach
Meadowbrook Lane
Staatsburg, NY 12580

I.R.A.
Att: Crew
P.O. Box 3
Centerville, MA 02632

Independence Rowing
Club
Thomas Kudzma
P.O. Box 1412
Nashua, NH 03061

Interlachen Rowing Club
P.O. Box 330
Corning, NY 14830

Iona College Crew
Dennis Lonergan
11 Irving Place
New Rochelle, NY 10801

Ithaca College Crew
Ceracche Center
Ithaca College
Ithaca, NY 14850

Kent School Boat Club
Kent School
Kent, CT 06757

Kings Crown Rowing
Assoc.
8 West 76th Street Apt A
New York, NY 10023

Lightweight Dev.
Camp/Club
Ms. K.C. Deitz
60 J.F. Kennedy Street
Cambridge, MA 02138

Little Brave Canoe
Rowing Club
Douglas E. Wood, MD
6 Whittier Place #4H
Boston, MA 02114

Manhattan College
Crew Club
Att: Athletic Dept.
Manhattan College
Bronx, NY 10471

Marist College
College Crew
McCann Center
Marist College
Poughkeepsie, NY 12601

Merrimack River
Rowing Assn.
500 Pawtucket Boulevard
Lowell, MA 01854

Middlesex School
Henry E. Erhard
Middlesex School
Concord, MA 01742

Middletown Rowing Assoc.
Middletown High School
Hunting Hill Avenue
Middletown, CT 06457

MIT Boat Club
Jane Betts
MIT Branch PO Box D
Cambridge, MA 02139

Monadnock Rowing Club
Att: Crew
P.O. Box 239
Harrisville, NH 03450

Mount Holyoke
Womens Regatta
Att: Crew
10 Harwich Place
South Hadley, MA 01075

Mount Madison
Vol. Ski Patrol
William Barrett
P.O. Box 78
JW McCormick Sta.
Boston, MA 02101

N.E.I.R.A.
Richard Davis
St. Paul's School
Concord, NH 03301

Narragansett Boat Club
PO Box 2413
Providence, RI 02906

New Haven Rowing Club
Norman Thetford
44 Collier Circle
Hamden, CT 06518

New York Athletic Club
F. X. Sulger
189 Sutton Manor
New Rochelle, NY 10805

Noble & Greenough
School
Att: Crew Coach
507 Bridge Street
Dedham, MA 02026

Nonesuch Oar & Paddle
Club
Phineas Sprague
Prouts Neck
Scarborough, ME 04074

Northeastern Univ. R.A.
Women's Ath. Dept.,
200 Arenx
360 Huntington Avenue
Boston, MA 02115

Northeastern University
Dept. of Athletics
360 Huntington Avenue
Boston, MA 02115

Northfield Mt. Hermon
School
Debbie Loomer
134 A French King Hwy.
Gill, MA 01376

NYSU—Maritime College
Att: Crew Coach
Fort Schuyler
Bronx, NY 10465

Oars
RD 1 Box 278
Voorheesville, NY 12186

Onota Lake Rowing Club
Peter Wells
PO Box 411
Williamstown, MA 01267

Pequot Yacht Club
George C. Wiswell, Jr.
130 Willow Street
Southport, CT 06490

Phillips Academy Crew
Att: Crew Coach
Phillips Academy
Andover, MA 01810

Pioneer Valley Rowing
Assoc.
Ferris Athletic Center
Trinity College
Hartford, CT 06106

Pomfret School
Andrew Washburn
Crew Coach
Pomfret, CT 06258

Porcellian Boat Club
John H. Canaday
PO Box 306
Exeter, NH 03833

Riverside Boat Club
Anne Noga
17 Kirkwood Rd.
Brighton, MA 02135

Rochester Rowing Club
Ronald Kwasman
41 Vick Park B
Rochester, NY 14607

Rude & Smooth Boat Club
Peter S. Lowe
46 East 91st Street
New York, NY 10028

Sagamore Rowing Assoc.
14 Windham Drive
Huntington Station
Long Island, NY 11746

Saint Mark's Boat Club
Crew Coach
St. Mark's School
Southborough, MA 01772

Salisbury Boat Club
Art Charles
Salisbury School
Salisbury, CT 06068

Salisbury Boat Club, Inc.
Richard Curtis
Emmons Lane
Canaan, CT 06018

Shimmo Rowing Club
Peter S. Heller
One Rockefeller Plaza
New York, NY 10020

Simsbury High School
Crew
Simsbury High School
34 Farms Village Road
Simsbury, CT 06092

Skidmore College
Attn: Crew
Ron Levene
Saratoga Springs, NY
12866

South Kent Crew
Att: Lawrence Smith
Crew Coach
South Kent School
South Kent, CT 06785

Sparhawk Sculling School
Peter Sparhawk
222 Porters Point Road
Colchester, VT 05446

Springfield College Crew
Chaplins Office
Springfield College
Springfield, MA 01109

Squamscott Scullers Inc.
Ernestine L. Bayer Jr.
371 Washington Road
Rye, NH 03870

St. John's University Crew
attn. Crew Coach
Union Tpke & Utopia Pkwy.
Jamaica NY 11432

St. John's High School
Att: Robert Foley
378 Main Street
Shrewsbury, MA 01545

St. Paul's School
Att: Crew
M.R. Blake
Concord, NH 03301

Syracuse Alumni Rowing
Assoc.
C. Roberts
P.O. Box 26
Lockport, NY 14094

Syracuse Chargers
Rowing Club
A. Carl Grantham, Pres.
4203 Mill Run Road
Liverpool, NY 13088

Syracuse University
Bill Sanford
Manley Field House
Syracuse, NY 13210

Tabor Academy
Rowing Assoc.
Att: Crew Coach
Front Street
Marion, MA 02738

The Gunnery School
Rick Malmstrom
The Gunnery School
Washington, CT 06793

The Tuxedo Rowing Club
Kurt S. Graetzer
50 E. Orchard Street
Allendale, NJ 07401

Trinity College
Burt Apfelbaum
Ferris Athletic Ctr.
Hartford, CT 06106

Tufts University
Ken Weinstein
Ath Dept/Tufts Univ.
Medford, MA 02155

U.S.C.G.A. CREW
Att: Crew Coach
U.S. Coast Guard Academy
New London, CT 06320

U.S.M.M.A. CREW
Att: Crew Coach
U.S. Merchant Marine
Academy
Kings Point, NY 11024

Union Boat Club
Att: Crew Coach
144 Chestnut Street
Boston, MA 02108

United Sports Assoc. R.C.
Att: Crew
395 E. Putnam Avenue
Cos Cob, CT 06807

Univ. of Connecticut
Crew Club
Brock Hall Box 223
77 Gilbert Road
Univ. of Conn.
Storrs, CT 06268

Univ. of Mass Rowing
Assoc.
Crew Office R. 9 NOPE
Univ. of Mass.
Amherst, MA 01002

Univ. of New Hampshire
Recreation Sports
151 Field House
Durham, NH 03824

Univ. of Rhode Island R.A.
Att: Head Coach/Crew
Rec. Off. Tootell Ctr., URI
Kingston, RI 02881

Univ. of Rochester Crew
Dept. of Sports &
Recreation
Zornow Ctr./Univ. of
Rochester
Rochester, NY 14627

University of Lowell Crew
University of Lowell
1 University Avenue
Lowell, MA 01854

Warren Rowing Club
Attn: Carlos Cordeiro
245 East 63rd Street
Apt 1516
New York, NY 10021

Wesleyan University
Donald M. Russel
Director of Athletics
Dept. of Phys. Education
Middletown, CT 06457

West Side Rowing Club
Att: Crew
217 Irving Terrace
Kenmore, NY 14223

Williams College Boat Club
P.O. Box 411
Williams College
Williamstown, MA 01267

Williamstown Boat Club
Att: Crew
P.O. Box 411
Williamstown, MA 01267

Winsor Crew
Margie McHugh
Pilgrim Road
Boston, MA 02215

Worcester Polytech R.A.
Crew Coach
WPI
Worcester, MA 01609

Worcester Rowing Assoc.
Thomas J. Sullivan
20 Old Colony Road
Shrewsbury, MA 01545

Yale University
402 A Yale Station
Athletic Dept.
New Haven, CT 06520

1980 Rowing Club
Holly Hatton
135 Lowell Street
Somerville, MA 02143

Mid-Atlantic

American Express
Rowing Assoc.
Sherry Hartigan
SE Cor. 16th & JFK
Philadelphia, PA 19102

American Rowing Assoc.
E.C.P. Thomas
16 Aldwyn Lane
Villanova, PA 19085

Bachelors Barge Club
Dr. Thomas Kerr, Jr.
116 E. Gorgas Lane
Philadelphia, PA 19119

Back Bay Viking Rowing
Club
Bob Garbutt
2 S. Rosborough Ave
Ventnor, NJ 08406

Baltimore Rowing Club
Howard Klein
PO Box 10162
Baltimore, MD 21285

Bonner Rowing Association
c/o Msgr Bonner HS
Landsdowne Avenue
and Garrett Road
Drexel Hill, PA 19026

Brigantine Rowing Club
Andrew A. Solari
705 Lafayette Blvd.
Brigantine, NJ 08203

Brooke High Crew Parents,
Inc.
Brooke High School
Cross Creek Road
Wellsburg, WV 26070

Bucknell Univ. Rowing Club
Box C 1057 Bucknell Univ.
Lewisburg, PA 17837

Camden County Rowing
Fdn.
William Knecht
P.O. Box 1346
Camden, NJ 08105

Camp Dimension
Charles P. Colgan
641 E. Shawmont Avenue
Phila., PA 19128

Carnegie Lake Rowing
Assoc.
Janet Spagnoli
55 Broadripple Drive
Princeton, NJ 08540

College Boat Club
Univ. of Pennsylvania
Bruce Konopka
33rd & Spruce Weightman
Hall
Philadelphia, PA 19104

Compote Rowing Assoc.
Dietrich Rose
4054 Ridge Avenue
Philadelphia, PA 19129

Crescent Boat Club
Att: Crew Coach
#5 Boathouse Row
Phila., PA 19130

Dad Vail Rowing Assoc.
Jack Seitz
1812 Webster Lane
Ambler, PA 19002

Drexel University Crew
Att: John Semanik
32nd & Chestnut Streets
Phila., PA 19104

Fairmount Rowing Assoc.
William J. Mastalski
877 N. Judson Street
Phila., PA 19130

Father Judge High School
Phillip Roche
5336 Saul Street
Phila., PA 19124

Fort Hunt High School
Att: Crew Coach
P.O. Box 6211
Alexandria, VA 22306

Garden State Games
Dick Steadman
16 Roosevelt Avenue
Deal, NJ 07723

George Mason Univ. Crew
Rm 251 Student Union 1
4400 University Drive
Fairfax, VA 22030

George Washington Univ.
Crew
Attn. Crew Coach
Dept. Intercoll. Athletics
Smith Street
Washington, DC 20056

Georgetown Univ. R.A.
Dept. of Athletics
Attn. Jay Forster
McDonough Arena
Washington, DC 20057

Holy Spirit High School
Rev. Michael D'Amico
Calif. & New Road
Absecon, NJ 08201

Hun School of Princeton
William Quirk, Athletic Dir.
PO Box 271
Princeton, NJ 08542

J.E.B. Stuart H.S.
Att: Crew Boosters
6319 Hillcrest Place
Alexandria, VA 22312

La Salle University Crew
20th & Olney Avenue
Philadelphia, PA 19141

La Salle College H.S.
Ken Shaw, Jr., Crew Coach
456 Militia Hill Road
Southampton, PA 18966

Lafayette College Crew
Club
Box 4140
Easton, PA 18042

Lehigh Valley Rowing
Assoc.
Steven B. Molder
340 Cattell Street
Easton, Pa 18042

Loyola College Crew Club
4501 N. Charles Street
Baltimore, MD 21210

Malta Boat Club
Ed Lentz
1049 Taylor Drive
Folcroff, PA 19032

Mary Washington Crew
Club
Box 3774 College Station
Fredericksburg, VA 22401

Mercyhurst College
Att: Crew Coach
501 E. 38th Street
Erie, PA 16546

Mercyhurst Prep School
Crew
Attn. Crew Coach
538 E. Grandview
Boulevard
Erie, PA 16504

Middle States R.A.
Joseph Hasiak
712 Monument Road
Malvern, PA 19355

Misery Bay Rowing Club
Stuart J. Miller
1324 So. Shore Drive
#904
Erie, PA 16505

Monongahela R.A. Inc.
Att: Crew Coach
P.O. Box 824
Morgantown, WV 26505

N.W.R.A.
Leisel Hud-Broderick
512 West Sedgewick
Philadelphia, PA 19119

National Rowing
Foundation
c/o Jack T. Franklin
P.O. Box 6030
Arlington, VA 22206

Navesink River Rowing
Club
Robert Verbrugge
100 Conover Place
Red Bank, NJ 07701

Northeast Catholic Crew
Sam Kahuila
#1 Willig
Philadelphia, PA 19125

Northern Virginia R.A
John Coffey
4220 25th Street
Arlington, VA 22207

Occoquan Boat Club
William Burruss
PO Box 5493
Springfield, VA 22150

Old Dominion B.C.
Dee Campbell
203 N. Ripley Street #303
Alexandria, VA 22304

Oneida Boat Club R.A.
c/o Corresponding Sect.
3 York Street
Burlington, NJ 08016

Penn Acad. R.A.
John T. Ervin, Treas.
5838 N. 4th Street
Philadelphia, PA 19120

Phila Frostbite Regatta
Coleman D. Boylan
#2 Boathouse Row
Philadelphia, PA 19130

Phila. Girls Rowing Club
Att: Captain
#14 Boathouse Row
Philadelphia, PA 19130

Potomac Boat Club
Secretary
3530 Water Street NW
Washington, DC 20007

Potomac Riv. Dev. Ctr.
John P. Devlin
1517 N. Taylor Street
Arlington, VA 22207

Prince Wm. Crew Assoc.,
Inc.
Woodbridge Chapter
P. O. Box 405
Occoquan, VA 22125

Princeton Univ. R.A.
Princeton Univ. (Crew)
Dept. of Athletics
Box 71
Princeton, NJ 08544

Provident National Bank
William Beldon
PO Box 7648
Philadelphia, PA 19101

Raritan Valley R.A.
Att: William T. Leavitt
P.O. Box 1149
Piscataway, NJ 08854

Regatta Sports
C. Read Murphy
16 West River Road
Rumson, NJ 07760

Rutgers Univ.
Att: William T. Leavitt
P.O. Box 1149
Piscataway, NJ 08854

Scholastic R.A.
Julian Whitestone
134 Sylvan Court
Alexandria, VA 22304

Schuylkill Navy
#4 Boathouse Row
East River Drive
Philadelphia, Pa 19130

Special Olympics
Rowing Program
James J. Wickersham
2826 Pickertown
Warrington, PA 18976

St. Andrew's School
Davis A. Washburn
Middletown, DE 19709

St. Joseph Prep R.A.
Charles Crawford
1009 Overbrook Road
Wilmington, DE 19807

Stockton St. College Crew
Att: Crew Coach
Stockton State College
Pomona, NJ 08240

T.C. Williams H.S.
c/o Don Riviere
3330 King Street
Alexandria, VA 22302

Temple University
Gavin White
3204 Brighton Street
Philadelphia, PA 19149

The Annapolis Rowing Club
Pat Guida
1031 Cedar Ridge Court
Annapolis, Maryland
21403

The Johns Hopkins Crew
White Athletics Center
Homewood,
Johns Hopkins Univ.
Baltimore, MD 21218

Trinity College Crew
Att: Crew Coach
Trinity College
Washington, DC 20017

Triton Boat Club
Att: Crew
24 Elmwood Avenue
Belleville, NJ 07109

U.S.N.A.
Crew
Att: Crew Coach
Annapolis, MD 21402

Undine Barge Club
John R. Oster
316 Kent Road
Wynnewood, PA 19096

Univ. Barge Cl;ub
c/o Secretary
#7 Boathouse Row
Philadelphia, PA 19130

Univ. of Penna.
Weightman Hall (Crew)
Dept. of Intercol. Athletics
Philadelphia, PA 19174

Univ. of Virginia R.A.
Memorial Gym.
Univ. of VA
Charlottesville, VA 22903

Univ. of Baltimore
Rowing Assoc.
Office of Student Activities
Charles St. &
Mt. Royal Avenue
Baltimore, MD 21211

Upper Merion B.C.
Phil Cavitt
125 Farmhouse Drive
Audobon, PA 19403

US Dragon Boat
Association
Ken Shaw, Jr.
456 Militia Hill Road
Southampton, PA 18966

Vesper Boat Club
Kirk Beckman
#10 Boat House Row
Phila., PA 19130

Viking Rowing Club
Stan Bergman
121 N. Oxford Avenue
Ventnor, NJ 08406

Gar-Field Crew Boosters
Club
Roger A Bolland
14203 N. Bismark Ave
Woodbridge, VA 22193

Villanova University
G. Tully Vaughan,
Head Coach
625 Bethlehem Park
Ambler, PA 19002

Washington & Lee H.S.
1300 No. Quincy Street
Arlington, VA 22201

Washington College Crew
Att: Crew Coach
Washington College
Chestertown, MD 21620

West Catholic
Rowing Assoc.
c/o John Cooke
2624 S. Shields Street
Philadelphia PA 19142

West River Rowing Club
Pat Anderson
2733 Fennel Road
Edgewater, MD 21037

Wharton Business Sch.
Rowing Assoc.
Peter Van Loan
111 Vance Hall, U. of Penn.
Philadelphia, PA 19104

Wilmington Rowing Club
PO Box 25248
Wilmington, DE 19899

Yorktown H.S. Crew
Al Villaret
5201 N. 28th Street
Arlington, VA 22207

YMCA Three Rivers Rowing
Assoc.
John Lubimer
3334 Benden Drive
Murrysville, PA 15668

Midwest

Austin Rowing Club
Att: Crew
1901 Travis Heights Blvd
Austin, TX 78704

Cincinnati Rowing Club
Harry H. Graves
2247 Spinningwheel Lane
Cincinnati, OH 45244

Creighton University Crew
Student Board of
Governors
Omaha, NE 68178

Culver Military/Girls Acad.
Attention Guy Weaser
Culver Military Acad./Bx 2
Culver, IN 46511

Des Moines Rowing Club,
Inc.
Ric. Jorgensen
4005 Kingman Boulevard
Des Moines, IA 50311

Detroit Boat Club
Richard Bell
27551 Rackham Drive
Lathrup Village, MI 48076

Duluth Rowing Club
Norine McVann
3614 Minnesota Avenue
Duluth, MN 55802

Friends of Detroit Rowing
c/o Gordon P. Hopman
6383 Vernmoor
Troy, MI 48098

Grand Valley Rowing Club
Bob Sawicki
9979 Bend Drive
Jenison, MI 49428

Indianapolis Boat Club, Inc.
PO Box 30339
Indianapolis, IN 46230

Iowa Rowing Association
Recreational Services
Field House
Iowa City, IA 52242

Kansas State Rowing
Assoc.
UPC/K-State Union
Kansas State University
Manhattan, KS 66506

Kansas University Crew
David Darwin
Dept. Civil Engineering
University of Kansas
Lawrence, KS 66045

Lincoln Park Boat Club
Gail Omohundro,
Secretary
511 West Melrose #306
Chicago, IL 60657

Macomb·YMCA
Rowing Program
Attn: K. Hadley
36691 Jefferson
Mt. Clemens, MI 48045

Marietta College Rowing
Assoc.
Att: Crew Coach
Marietta College
Marietta, OH 45750

Mendota Rowing Club
PO Box 646
Madison, WI 53701

Michigan State Univ. Crew
231 I.M. West
Michigan State Univ.
East Lansing, MI 48824

Milwaukee Rowing Club,
Inc.
Milwaukee Rowing Club
5335 N. Diversey
Boulevard
Milwaukee, WI 53217

Minneapolis Rowing Club
PO Box 6712
Minneapolis, MN 55406

Minnesota Boat Club
1 So Wabasha St/Navy Is.
St. Paul, MN 55107

Nebraska Univ. Crew
Att: Crew Program
1000 N. 16th Street
Lincoln, NE 68588

Northwestern Univ. Crew
Patten Gymnasium
2407 Sheridan Road
Evanston, IL 60201

Notre Dame Rowing Club
PO Box 55
Notre Dame, IN 46556

Ohio State University Crew
Jeffrey H. Houston H.C.
223 W. 8th Avenue
Columbus, OH 43201

Oklahoma City
Rowing Club
P.O. Box 1937
Oklahoma City, OK 73101

Purdue Crew Club
Co-Recreational Gym
Purdue University
W. Lafayette, IN 47906

Sooner Rowing Assoc.
Charles W. Oliphant
4400 One Williams Center
Tulsa, OK 74172

St Louis Rowing Club
PO Box 16292
St. Louis, MO 63105

Texas Crew
Rec. Sports, U. of Texas
Gregory Gym 33
Austin, TX 78712

Toledo Rowing Club
Jerry Brown, President
5771 Bay Shore Road
Oregon, OH 43616

Toledo Rowing Foundation
Steven W. Monro
Monro Steel
8201 W. Central Avenue
Toledo, OH 43617

Topeka Rowing Association
Don Craig
4336 SE 25th Street
Terrace
Topeka, KS 66605

University of Chicago
Women's Crew
Susan K. B. Urbas
400 E. Randolph Street
#2527
Chicago, IL 60601

Univ. of Chicago
Coed Crew
c/o Ian Sweedler
1154 E 56th Street #4
Chicago, IL 60637

Univ. of Michigan
Rowing Club
North Campus Rec. Bldg.
Univ. of Michigan
Ann Arbor, MI 48109

University of MN
Women's Crew
238 Bierman Building
516 15th Avenue SE
Minneapolis, MN 55455

University of Minnesota
Crew
Men's Crew Program
107 Norris Hall
Minneapolis, MN 55455

Univ. of Wisconsin Crew
Att: Crew Coach
1440 Monroe Street
Madison, WI 53706

Waterloo Rowing Club
Att: Crew Program
P.O. Box 1435
Waterloo, IA 50704

Wayne State Univ. Crew
Div. of Health & Phys. Ed.
Wayne State University
Detroit, MI 48202

Wichita State Univ. Crew
137 N. Waco
Wichita, KS 67202

Wyndotte Boat Club
Att: Crew Coach
P.O. Box 341
Wyndotte, MI 48192

Xavier University Crew
Graham Coles
5695 Valley Forge Drive
Fairfield, OH 45014

Ecorse Rowing Club
4496 High Street Apt #4
Ecorse, MI 48229

Chicago Aquatic Center
Susan K.B. Urbas
400 E. Randolph Street
#2527
Chicago, IL 60601

Southeast

Academia Cubana de
Remo
Att: Crew
P.O. Box 592812
Miami, FL 33159

AFG Rowing Club
Mark Ford
1000 University Blvd D-6
Kingsport, TN 37660

American Barge Club, Inc.
Aldo F. Berti, M.D.
1321 NW 14th Street
Suite 214
Miami, FL 33136

Atlanta Rowing Club, Inc.
Gordon Hunter
14680 Wood Road
Alpharetta, GA 30201

Augusta Rowing Club
Cobbs Nixon
641 Broad Street
Augusta, GA 30901

Bulldog Rowing Club
James J. Millar
701 Oxford
Houston, TX 77007

Charleston Rowing Club
Att: Crew
University of Charleston
Charleston, WV 25304

Dallas Rowing Club
PO Box 7309
Dallas, TX 75209

Augusta Port Authority
C. Thompson Harley
Box 2084
Augusta, GA 30903

Duke Men's Crew
PO Box 9150 Duke Station
Durham, NC 27706

Edgewater High School
Martyn Dennis
1324 Indiana Avenue
Winter Park, FL 32789

Florida Athletic Club
c/o John R. Ingram
401 E. Tullis Avenue
Longwood, FL 32750

Florida Inst. of Tech.
Wm. K. Jurgens
POB 1150, Athletic Dept.
Melbourne, FL 32901

Governor's Council
Phys. Fitness & Sports
Office of the Governor
The Capitol
Tallahassee, FL 32301

Harbor City Rowing Club
Billie K. Brown
2900 Riverview Drive
Melbourne, FL 32901

Jacksonville Episcopal
High School Crew
Arthur Peterson, Head
Coach
4455 Atlantic Boulevard
Jacksonville, FL 32207

Jacksonville Univ. Crew
Att: Crew Coach
2800 Univ. Boulevard
North
Jacksonville, FL 32211

Knoxville Rowing Assoc.
P.O. Box 138
Knoxville, TN 37901

Lookout Rowing Club
c/o Newton Cheverolet
W. M. L. King & Riverfront
Chattanooga, TN 37402

Miami Rowing Club
P.O. Box 593061
Miami, FL 33159

Oak Ridge Rowing Assoc.
P.O. Box 75
Oak Ridge, TN 37831

Palm Beach Rowing Assoc.
James K. Green
301 Clematis Street
Suite 200
West Palm Beach, FL
33401

Palm Beach Rowing Club
Edward I. Singer
1460 S. Ocean Boulevard
Lantana, FL 33462

Remex Rowing Club, Inc.
5403 Oliver Street No.
Jacksonville, FL 32211

Rollins College
Attn. Crew
P.O. Box 2730
Winter Park, FL 32789

S.I.R.A.
Norton Schlachter, Pres.
2729 St. Augustine Trail
Marietta, GA 30067

St. John's Few Rowing Club
c/o Kristen Negaard Dees
763 Egret Bluff Lane
Jacksonville, FL 32211

Tampa Rowing Club
Jorge Rodriguez
4712 Estrella
Tampa, FL 33629

The Citadel Crew
Att: Crew Coach
Dept. of Physical Ed.
Charleston, SC 29409

Univ. of No. Carolina Crew
Mark Pavao
Box 16, Carolina Union
Chapel Hill, NC 27514

Univ. of Al. in Huntsville
Att: Crew Team
Univ. of Alabama
Huntsville, AL 35899

Univ. of Tenn. R.C.
Dave Brownell, Pres.
2106 Andy Holt/
Student Aquat. Ctr.
Knoxville, TN 37916

Vista Shores Rowing Crew
Raoul P. Rodriguez
741 Robert E. Lee
Boulevard
New Orleans, LA 70124

Winter Park High School
Att: Rowing Club
2100 Summerfield Road
Winter Park, FL 32789

Wolf River Rowing Club
Kemper B. Durand
44 N. Second Street 9th Fl
Memphis, TN 38103

Southwest

Berkeley Crew Club
C. Lynn Cary
1224 Oxford Street
Berkeley, CA 94709

Calif. Maritime Academy
Att: Crew Coach
Maritime Academy Drive
Vallejo, CA 94590

Calif. Univ. of Irvine
Att: Crew Coach
Dept. of Athletics
Irvine, CA 92717

Calif. Univ. of Los Angeles
Att: Crew Coach
405 Hilgard Avenue
Los Angeles, CA 90024

Calif. Univ. of San Diego
Att: Crew Coach
PE Dept. S-005
La Jolla, CA 92093

Calif. Yacht Club
Att: Crew
4469 Admiralty Way
Marina del Rey, CA 90291

California Rowing Club
Ky Ebright Boathouse
2909 Glascock Street
Oakland, CA 94601

Golden Bear Rowing
Association
Nanette Bernadou
2415 College Avenue #14
Berkeley, CA 94704

Graham Recreational
Rowers
R.E. Graham
P.O. Box 2278
Orange, CA 92669

Lake Merritt Rowing Club
Att: Crew
P.O. Box 1046
Oakland, CA 94604

Long Beach Rowing Assoc.
Att: Crew
P.O. Box 3879
Long Beach, CA 90803

Los Gatos Rowing Club
Att: Crew
22025 Old Santa Cruz
Highway
Los Gatos, CA 95030

Loyola Marymount R.A.
Att: Crew Coach
7101 W. 80th Street
Los Angeles, CA 90045

Marin Rowing Assoc.
Mrs Joan Corbett,
Secretary
490 Riviera Circle
Larkspur, CA 94939

Mission Bay Rowing Assoc.
Att: Executive Director
1001 Santa Clara Place
San Diego, CA 92109

Motley Rowing Club
James Willis
256B Newport Ave.
Long Beach, CA 90803

Newport Beach R.C.
Brad Lewis
505 Begonia Avenue
Corona del Mar, CA
92625

Oakland Strokes
Ed Lickiss
4419 Moraga Avenue
Oakland, CA 94611

Orange Coast College
Rowing Assc.
Attn. David Grant
2701 Fairview Road
Costa Mesa, CA 92626

River City Rowing Club
Merri Lisa Formento
2816 Land Park Drive
Sacramento, CA 95818

San Diego Rowing Club
P.O. Box 2768
San Diego, CA 92112

San Francisco Police
Athletic Club
Mark E. Hurley
366 Mississippi Street
San Francisco, CA 94107

Santa Clara Univ. R.A.
Att: Crew Coach
Santa Clara Univ.
Santa Clara, CA 95053

St. Mary's College Crew
Giancarlo Trevisan
15945 Via Cordoba
San Lorenzo, CA 94580

Stanford Drew Association
Stanford University
Athletic Dept.
Stanford, CA 94305

Stockton Rowing Club
P.O.B. 2181
Stockton, CA 95201

The Dirty Dozen
Allen H. Trant
4 Commodore #328
Emeryville, CA 94608

UC Davis Crew
140 Recreation Hall
U.C. Davis
Davis, CA 95616

Univ. of So. Calif. Crew
Heritage Hall, Dept of Ath.
University Park
Los Angeles, CA 90089

University of Calif.,
Berkeley
Men's Intercol. Athletics-
Crew
Harmon Gym, Univ. of CA
Berkeley, CA 94720

Western Intercol. Rowing
Assn.
Morris H. Lax
2611 Corona Drive
Davis, CA 95616

ZLAC Rowing Club
Att: CREW
1111 Pacific Beach Drive
San Diego, CA 92109

Northwest

Anchorage Navy
Robert E. Miller
7729 Anne Circle
Anchorage, AK 99504

Bush School Crew
Tom Jordan, Coach
405 36th Avenue E
Seattle, WA 98112

Deschutes Rowing Club
Meg Fraser
200 Pacific Park Lane
Bend, OR 97701

Everett Rowing Assoc.
Junior Rowing
Martin D. Beyer
2210 Baker Avenue
Everett, WA 98201

Gonzaga University
Rowing Assoc.
Rev. Michael Siconolfi, S.J.
Jesuit Hous
Gonzaga Univ.
Spokane, WA 99258

Green Lake Crew
Seattle Dept. Parks/Rec.
100 Dexter Avenue North
Seattle, WA 98109

Humboldt State Univ. R.A.
P.O. Box 393
Arcata Ca 95521

Lake Ewauna Rowing Club
Lois L. Robinson
2604 Wiard Street
Klamath Falls, OR 97603

Portland Rowing Club
Laurel Lynn Anderson
5723 NE Skidmore Apt 5
Portland, OR 97218

Lake Washington
Rowing Club
PO Box 45117
University Station
Seattle, WA 98145

Lakeside School
Att: Crew Coach
14050 First Avenue NE
Seattle, WA 98125

Lute Varsity Rowing Club
Att: Crew
Athletic Dept. PLU
Tacoma, WA 98447

OIT Rowing Club
College Union Bldg.
Klamath Falls, OR 97601

Oregon State
Rowing Assoc.
103 Gill Coliseum
Oregon State University
Corvallis, OR 97331

Overlake School
Att: Crew Coach
20301 NE 108th
Redmond, WA 98052

Seattle Pacific Crew
Att: Crew Coach
Seattle Pacific University
Seattle, WA 98119

Seattle Tennis Club
Hugh C. Klopfenstein
922 McGilvra Blvd. E.
Seattle, WA 98122

George Y. Pocock
Rowing Center
Alan Mackenzie, DDS
2109 Whitman NE
Renton, WA 98056

Station L Rowing Club
Michael G. Roehr
654 N. E. Royal Court
Portland, OR 97232

Union Bay Rowing Club
Univ. of Washington
Sports Clubs GD-10
Seattle, WA 98195

Univ. of Puget Sound
Att: Crew Coach
1500 N. Warner Street
Tacoma, WA 98416

Univ. of Washington
Crew House
Univ. of WA - GC-20
Seattle, WA 98195

University of Oregon
Att: Crew Coach
EMU Club Sports
Eugene, OR 97403

Washington State
University
Cougar Crew
3rd Floor CUB
Pullman, WA 99164

Western Washington
University
Fil Leanderson, Coach
OM 365 - WWU
Bellingham, WA 98225

Wilamette Rowing Club
Frank Zagunis
55 SW Oriole Lane
Lake Oswego, OR 97034

About the Authors

Professionals from several disciplines, but with a common interest in physical fitness, have designed a balanced program of strength and endurance training using these machines. They include:

Barbara Kirch, who has outlined the techniques of rowing and offers instruction on how to avoid rowing-related injuries. She was a member of the U.S. national rowing team in 1982, captain of the Pennsylvania women's rowing team in 1983, and a member of the U.S. Olympic rowing team in 1984. She has also rowed with the Vespers Boat Club, a prestigious Philadelphia rowing organization, and The Hamburger Ruderinnen Club in Hamburg, where she trained with members of the West German national rowing team. A graduate of the University of Pennsylvania, she plans on pursuing a career in physical therapy and athletic training.

Dr. Reed W. Hoyt, an exercise physiologist who has studied long-distance runners and elite rowers, designed the program so that endurance, with improved heart and lung function, and strength, with attendant muscle development, can be achieved. A practical guide to nutrition helps the reader choose a diet compatible with the goals of his or her particular exercise program. Staffs of several cardiac rehabilitation centers have confirmed the positive benefits of exercise with these machines.

Dr. Hoyt is affiliated with the Division of Hematology at The Children's Hospital of Philadelphia. He has done studies on elite rowers to evaluate the effectiveness of their training, and the physiologic basis of extraordinary athletic performance. He is also studying the role of exercise in children with chronic anemia.

Janet Fithian, a medical writer, through an examination of the medical literature, conversations with experts, and personal experience, is convinced that the home rowing machine is a safe, enjoyable, and effective form of exercise. She is writer/editor for the Division of Hematology at The Children's Hospital in Philadelphia, where she prepares patient education materials, writes proposals and reports, and edits scientific papers. She is author of *Understanding the Child with a Chronic Illness in the Classroom*. As a freelance writer she has placed articles with *Parents, American Baby, Better Homes, Seventeen,* and the *Denver Post Sunday Supplement*.